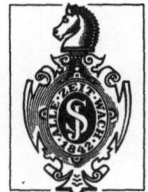

Edgar W. Somerville

Displacement of the Hip in Childhood

Aetiology, Management and Sequelae

With 262 Figures

Springer-Verlag
Berlin Heidelberg New York 1982

Edgar W. Somerville, MA, FRCS, FRCS(Ed)

Emeritus Consultant in Orthopaedics
The Nuffield Orthopaedic Centre
Oxford, England

ISBN-13:978-1-4471-1313-3   e-ISBN-13:978-1-4471-1311-9
DOI: 10.1007/978-1-4471-1311-9

Library of Congress Cataloging in Publication Data
Somerville, Edgar W. (Edgar William), 1913–   Displacement of the Hip in Child-
hood, Aetiology, Management, and Sequelae. Includes bibliographies and index. 1. Hip
joint—Dislocation. 2. Hip joint—Dislocation, Congenital. 3. Pediatric orthopedia.
I. Title. [DNLM: 1. Hip dislocation—In infancy and childhood. WE 860 S696d]
RD 772.S65 617′. 397 81–9355
ISBN-13:978-1-4471-1313-3 (U.S.) AACR2

© by Springer-Verlag Berlin Heidelberg 1982
Softcover reprint of the hardcover 1st edition 1982

Typeset by Phoenix Photosetting Chatham

2128/3916–543210

I wish to dedicate this book
to my wife Margaret

Contents

Preface

This book is concerned with the effect that displacement, whether minimal or severe, may have on the hip joint. Although it is concerned with the changes which take place in childhood and during growth, when they are most common and most severe, it is also to a lesser extent concerned with the way they will continue or even start long after growth has ceased.

It is based on a series of about 450 cases of congenital displacement of the hip treated when the deformity was established, together with unstable hips drawn from 82 000 children whose hips were examined at the time of birth.

This study was carried out at the Nuffield Orthopaedic Centre in Oxford. It was started in early 1949 by the author with Mr. J. C. Scott and continued until mid-1977, since when it has continued in the capable hands of Mr. J. W. Goodfellow and Mr. M. K. Benson.

The study was started at a time when the generally accepted view was still that the displacement was part of the primary failure of development of the acetabulum, which could not adequately contain the femoral head. Conservative treatment with manipulative reduction followed by a prolonged period of plaster immobilisation was the method of choice. Few attempts had been made with surgery as a primary procedure and these had not met with continuing success.

The concept on which this study was based was that the hip which became displaced was basically normal and that the changes seen in established displacement were all secondary to the displacement. The displacement occurred at or about the time of birth as a result of stresses applied to a temporarily softened capsule. The idea was that if these secondary changes were corrected definitively by surgery so that normal mechanics were restored to the joint in time, the hip should be able to develop normally while being used in a normal manner. The method of treatment described in this book has remained the same throughout apart from two minor changes—division of the transverse acetabular ligament routinely and the addition of 15° of varus to the rotation osteotomy—both of which were included during the last 8 or 9 years. It was inevitable, since there was little previous work along these lines to act as a guide, that errors would be made. These were usually the result of a mistaken urge to be more conservative. Operations were delayed or were inadequate, leading to a number of failures which necessitated second operations to do what should have been done properly the first time.

In 1957, with the full co-operation of Dr. Victoria Smallpiece and Dr. Hugh Ellis, the paediatricians at the Radcliffe Infirmary, routine examination of the hips of all new-born children at the Oxford hospitals was started. This was later extended to the periphery through lectures in hospitals and instruction to general practitioners and midwives.

Also in 1957, the minor displacement so often seen in Perthes' disease seemed to take on a greater significance. It was found that this could quite easily be reduced and the reduction maintained by a suitable high femoral osteotomy, with a surprising degree of remodelling taking place over a period of many years. These cases have been treated surgically ever since, and experience with the technique is described.

Throughout the whole of these series it has become increasingly apparent how readily the development of the hip joint can be influenced, for better or for worse, by alterations in the mechanics. While this is more obvious in young children, in whom the changes take place rapidly, it also occurs in any age group, though more slowly as age advances. It is this theme of the malleability of joints in the presence of mechanical changes, even though they may be very small, which is the basis of this book.

Oxford, June 1981   Edgar W. Somerville

Acknowledgements: I would like to acknowledge the great help and support I received from Mr. J. C. Scott, who played a large part in the early days and was responsible for the introduction of the frame as a means of reducing the displacement without trauma, which did more than anything else to reduce the incidence of osteochondritis.

I wish also to acknowledge the support of all my colleagues both at the Nuffield Orthopaedic Centre and at the peripheral hospitals, who did me the honour of referring their patients to me, and that of the paediatricians at the Radcliffe Infirmary, with whom I had such a happy and useful relationship in the early diagnosis of hip displacement.

For more than 28 years I was fortunate in having with me many excellent residents, many of whom contributed to this concept, and particularly Mr. G. P. Mitchell, now of Edinburgh, who was particularly involved in the early years and has added so much on his own since.

The treatment of the cases referred to here cannot be undertaken without a highly efficient nursing staff. I was indeed fortunate in having the help first of Sister Martin for 15 years and then of Sister Howard for 13. Without their invaluable help I do not think this work could ever have been done. At the same time I can never forget the help I received from the after-care Sisters, the theatre staff, and all those concerned with the outpatient clinics.

The follow-up of such a large number of patients, all with visual and written records maintained up to date all the time, involves a great deal of work. I was most fortunate in having Mrs. Joan Anderson as my Secretary for many years. I very much doubt whether such a follow-up could have been achieved without her tremendous enthusiasm.

I would like to acknowledge the great help I received from all members of the Photographic Department under the care of Mr. Bob Emmanuel, and I am most grateful to Mr. Anthony Rollason, the surgical artist, for the drawings he did for me (Figs. 5.32, 5.52, and 8.9).

I am most grateful for the help I have received from Mr. J. Crawford Adams in the writing of this book. I greatly appreciated his constructive and helpful advice.

Lastly I would like to thank the patients and their parents, who so loyally continued to attend the special C.D.H. clinic, often at great inconvenience to themselves, often long after they could see any good reason for doing so; in doing so they made such a long follow-up a practical possibility.

A great deal of what appears in this book has been previously recorded in papers to journals, chiefly the *Journal of Bone and Joint Surgery* (British edition), and I am grateful to the Editor for permission to reproduce a number of the illustrations. I am also grateful to the Editors of the *Proceedings of the Royal Society of Medicine* and the *Israeli Journal of Surgery* for permission to reproduce illustrations and tables which have appeared in these journals, and to the Editor of *Acta Orthopaedica Belgica* for permission to include illustrations in the section on Perthes' disease which originally appeared in his symposium.

1 Aetiology

The nomenclature of diseases has always presented a problem, to which no satisfactory solution has so far been found. Some diseases have been named after those thought to have been the first to describe them. This led to difficulties because of uncertainty as to who really had first described a condition, and sometimes the same disease has been called by different names in different countries. Others have been named according to the supposed pathology, but sometimes increasing knowledge suggests a different pathology. The name is then wrong but is firmly established in the literature and will be actually misleading.

In the case of other conditions, of which congenital dislocation of the hip is one, it may become apparent that the name by which it is generally known may cover a number of lesions which have little in common. In such circumstances the pathological changes in one lesion may be mistakenly assumed to be the same in another, leading to a misunderstanding of its true nature.

In the many different types of dislocation of the hip in infancy the only common feature is the dislocation. The displacement may have occurred in any of a number of different ways, making the nature of each lesion, and often the method of correction, quite different. The fact that at present they are all accorded the same name leads to confusion and misunderstanding of the underlying pathology.

Dislocation of the hip in infancy may result from the effect of muscle imbalance, from the presence of congenital contractures, from intrauterine compression, from true teratological abnormalities or from factors which are suspected but still unproved.

In the first four types the dislocation is only a minor incident in a far more serious disease, and only in the last is the dislocation a disease entity in itself with nothing else wrong with the child. This last type has been called 'typical congenital dislocation of the hip' (Hass 1948) and is the type usually meant by the term 'congenital dislocation of the hip'. Unfortunately the pathology of other types is often identified with this type without adequate justification.

PATHOLOGY

No other animal has a hip that is similar to that of man, and because of these anatomical differences it is unlikely that the study of animal hips will provide useful information that will extend our understanding of pathological changes in this joint.

Since there is no 'test bed' from which information as to the nature of congenital dislocation of the hip can be obtained, the only source of information available is obtained from the study of many hips in children, in health and in disease, throughout the period of growth.

The source of the information given in this monograph has been the study of some

400 patients with established displacement of the hip, followed up at regular intervals for up to 25 years after treatment, and conditions such as persistent foetal
alignment of the femoral neck, congenital coxa vara, and vascular and growth
changes in the upper end of the femur, as in Perthes' disease.

It is apparent that ossification and bone growth are dependent upon blood supply.
Wherever an ossific nucleus develops there must be an artery and a vein; the growth
of the nucleus is dependent on the maintenance of this blood supply, but the speed of
growth is greatly influenced by the stresses to which the bone is subjected. Wolff's
law states that development is directly proportional to the stresses applied to the
bone. If stress is reduced, as in paralysis or instability, ossification will be retarded.
Stress also has a marked effect on the shape of the bone or joint. The final shape
depends not only on the initial shape of the cartilaginous anlage but also on the
stresses to which it is subjected during growth. A growing bone subjected to normal
stress will grow into a shape which has come to be considered as normal, but if it is
subjected to some different stress it will develop into a different shape. This ability of
bones and joints to be modelled by the stresses and strains to which they are exposed
is very great, and is far greater and continues much longer than is commonly
supposed, so that the purpose of any form of treatment must be directed towards the
establishment of normal mechanics. Without this no bone or joint can develop
normally during the period of growth, and it is likely that after growth has ceased the
same phenomenon will continue, but at a slower rate.

It is important to differentiate between deformities due to abnormalities of
growth, which will keep on recurring after correction, and those due to faulty
mechanics, which will progressively correct themselves once the mechanical defect
has been corrected.

Armed with this simple knowledge, it is possible to go some way towards determining the way in which displacement occurs and the nature of the structural deformities
which develop later.

Cause of Displacement

ACETABULAR DYSPLASIA

There has long been a belief that primary dysplasia is either the cause of the
displacement or plays a large part in it, but the available evidence is against this.

It is known that at the time of birth instability of the hip or frank displacement of
the head of the femur is not uncommon, but by the end of the first week of life in
60%–70% (Barlow 1966) of these cases the joint has become stable spontaneously
without treatment, and in the 30%–40% in which instability persists simple splintage
in the reduced position for a few months restores normality.

If some instablity persists after 2 years, which is very uncommon, it can readily be
corrected by a suitable femoral oesteotomy (p. 23) restoring normal mechanics to
the joint. Only if the displacement is allowed to persist will secondary structural
changes develop. It is these secondary changes which have so often been mistakenly
assumed to be primary ones. These facts strongly suggest that there is no primary
acetabular defect.

CAPSULAR LAXITY

The stability of joints depends on the integrity of the soft tissues rather than on the
shape of the joint surfaces.

Capsular laxity can take two forms: Firstly the laxity of the whole of the capsule, which allows an increased range of movement in all directions but not necessarily displacement. Such capsular laxity may not be a cause of displacement but there is no doubt that where severe generalised laxity exists correction of a dislocated hip may prove very difficult and the prognosis may be poor. Dislocated hips associated with severe degrees of Ehlers–Danlos disease are probably better left alone. The importance of such capsular laxity has been appreciated for many years, since it was described by Le Damany (1905), and more recently by Carter and Wilkinson (1964).

Secondly, laxity as the result of stretching may develop in a part of the capsule, while the rest remains normal or even contracted. It is in this type of laxity that displacement is more likely to occur.

Andren (1960, 1962) suggested that capsular laxity might be caused by the effect of the maternal relaxing hormones present in the bloodstream at birth, and that this might well affect the ligaments of the child's joints before, during, and after birth for a short time. He was able to demonstrate laxity of the ligaments in certain newborn infants, Wilkinson (1963) showed the relaxant effect of oestrogen injected into young rabbits, which made the displacement of the hips easier, and Andren and Borglin (1961) showed a possible anomaly in oestrogen metabolism in newborn children with instability of the hips. But in spite of this, the nature of the displacement is still uncertain because there never has been any confirmation of a true hormonal imbalance of a temporary nature in the neonatal period, and Ruth Wynne-Davies (1970), following an extensive review, considers that this is unlikely to be the cause of displacement.

In spite of this there are several factors which make the theory attractive, because they fit in with the known facts:

1) It is beyond doubt that the capsule is stretched in the congenitally displaced hip, whether dislocated or subluxated, because the head remains within it, whereas in traumatic displacement the capsule is ruptured.

2) The capsule in a normal hip at birth is a strong structure, and attempts at dislocation in the stillborn child result in fracture of the femur rather than displacement of the hip. It seems that the capsule must be abnormally stretchable in those children who are at risk.

3) Whatever it is that causes the weakening of the capsule must have only a transient effect, because of the strong tendency for the instability to resolve spontaneously in the first week of life in the great majority of cases and the ease with which the rest respond to treatment. This could only happen if the laxity were a temporary phenomenon.

It is difficult to think of anything which fits the facts better than the hormonal hypothesis.

POSITION

It has been suggested, with much justification, that the position of the femur has an effect on the development of displacement. Weissman (1954) suggested that adduction of the hip in the infant was at least a contributory factor in displacement. He suggested that the adduction was really the result of an abduction deformity of the opposite hip. This is certainly the case in paralytic dislocation of the hip occurring in young children with poliomyelitis (Somerville 1959). Lloyd-Roberts and Swann (1966) described the condition of pelvic obliquity in infancy, as a result of which one hip was persistently adducted. This condition is not usually discovered until some months after birth, when the decision as to whether to treat or not may be very difficult to make. The appearance strongly suggests that the hip may be damaged if the deformity is allowed to persist, and indeed Weissman (1954) has reported that in a series of 51, two children developed dislocations. There is, however, some risk in undertaking treatment by wide abduction. Lloyd-Roberts has pointed out the risk involved in splinting these hips in abduction if any force is used. This risk cannot be taken lightly, because the damage which may be done to the blood supply to the head will lead to deformities which are severe and irreversible. For this reason the present author, when he has treated this condition, has applied a soft cushion to prevent adduction rather than to produce abduction. There is no certainty that the hip requires more than careful watching. In the small number seen none has come to harm.

INTRAUTERINE COMPRESSION

The damage that can be done to the foetus by intrauterine compression was first emphasised by Dennis Browne (1936) and later by Dunn (1969, 1976). They showed the great damage that can be done to the foetus in this way, including dislocation of the hips. They considered that in milder cases pressure on the flexed knee could cause displacement of the hip without other obvious damage to the child and that this was the cause of congenital dislocation of the hip.

Time of Displacement

It is apparent that at the time of birth many hips are unstable but there is a strong tendency to spontaneous resolution and a ready response to treatment. A deformity which has been present in utero for some time before birth is likely to be difficult to treat, because of the development of contractures and even secondary structural changes before the child is born. The ease with which these hips can be corrected suggests that the displacement is of recent origin, possibly having happened during the process of birth, possibly soon after, and not associated with more than minimal trauma.

There is also a possibility that displacement may develop gradually in the months after birth. If displacement occurs late it is likely that it will be of a minor degree rather than a complete dislocation.

Direction of Displacement

As already mentioned it seems likely that displacement occurs as a result of stretching of the previously weakened capsule and that it is a part of the capsule that is stretched rather than the whole.

In the literature there are descriptions of the displacement occurring posteriorly, superiorly, inferiorly and anteriorly, each direction being associated with a different mechanism. Again it is only possible to resolve the different views in the light of the known facts, since there is no animal available in which the human hip can be simulated.

POSTERIOR

The most commonly accepted view has been that the dislocation takes place posteriorly. This is based on the very obvious fact that when manipulative reduction is carried out the head of the femur is reduced over the posterior lip of the acetabulum into the joint, and that in old-established dislocations which come to necropsy there is a marked deficiency of the posterior lip of the acetabulum, through which it is believed the displacement took place (Fig. 1.1).

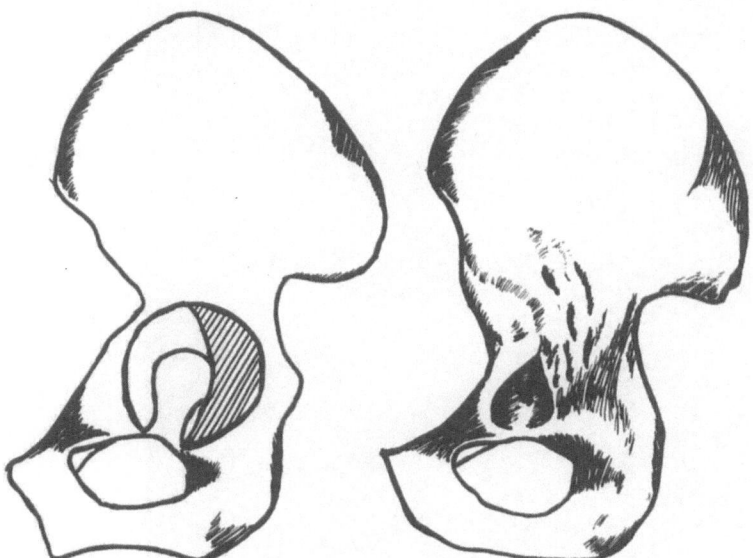

Fig. 1.1. The drawing on the *right* is of a specimen in the museum of the Royal College of Surgeons in London. It shows the acetabulum in an old untreated dislocation of the hip. Posteriorly there is a bony ledge overlapping the posterior half of the acetabulum. The drawing on the *left* depicts a normal acetabulum, with the *shaded area* showing the area covered by a typical inverted limbus. There is a strong suggestion that the ledge on the right is an inverted limbus which has become ossified. (See also Fig. 1.5)

Examination of the established dislocated hip in a child in whom the flexion contracture present at birth has been corrected will show the femoral head just below and lateral to the anterior superior iliac spine, from which it must be distinguished, when the hip is in extension. If the hip is flexed to 90° the femoral head can be felt to pass posteriorly. This can also be demonstrated radiologically (Fig. 1.2).

Since flexing the hip to 90° is an integral part of manipulative reduction it is not surprising that the femoral head is reduced over the posterior lip of the acetabulum.

Subluxation can be reduced by simple medial rotation with the hip in extension, because subluxations are always anterior.

To postulate that dislocation takes place posteriorly it must be assumed that subluxation and dislocation are two different conditions. To postulate that subluxation and dislocation are the same condition and that the difference is simply a matter of degree implies that the direction of displacement must initially be anterior. This would be incompatible with displacement before birth but consistent with displacement immediately after birth when the hips are extended for the first time.

INFERIOR

Displacement inferiorly has been suggested, and this would be consistent with the

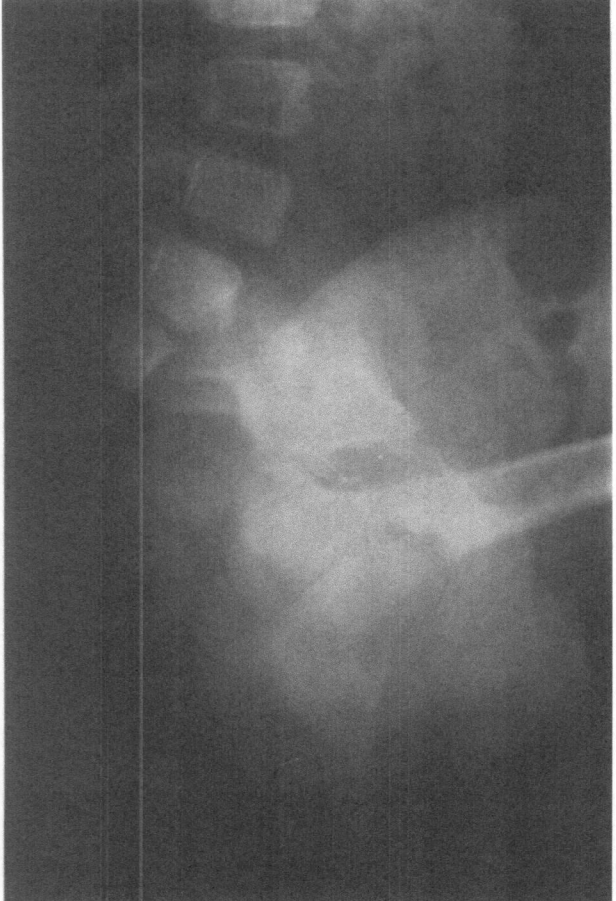

Fig. 1.2. Lateral radiograph of the pelvis of a child with bilateral dislocations, with one hip in extension and the other flexed. In extension the head is anterior, in flexion it is posterior

fact that displacement is commoner in breech presentations, in which the direction of thrust would be expected to be downwards.

The danger of placing the hips of the newborn child in wide abduction is becoming increasly apparent, and it has been suggested (Salter 1970; Trevor 1972) that in the child a few months old at the time of diagnosis the hips should be flexed to 90° but only abducted to about 30°. This position has been called the 'human position', because of its resemblance to the foetal position in utero. Since this is a safe position and maintains a good reduction it seems to be extremely unlikely that displacement occurs through the notch inferiorly in any but the most exceptional cases, because it would be against all common sense to place the limb in the position in which the displacement took place in order to keep it reduced.

ANTERIOR

It is often inferred that displacement occurs in an upward and outward direction. This is the result of the radiological appearance which, if taken at its face value, suggests that this is the case. Examination of the child and a critical examination of the x-ray plates shows that the head of the femur leaves the acetabulum anteriorly with lateral rotation and can be replaced by medial rotation (Figs. 1.3 and 1.4). Furthermore, as already mentioned, subluxations are always anterior, so that if dislocations are not anterior dislocation and subluxation must be two different conditions, which seems ·very unlikely.

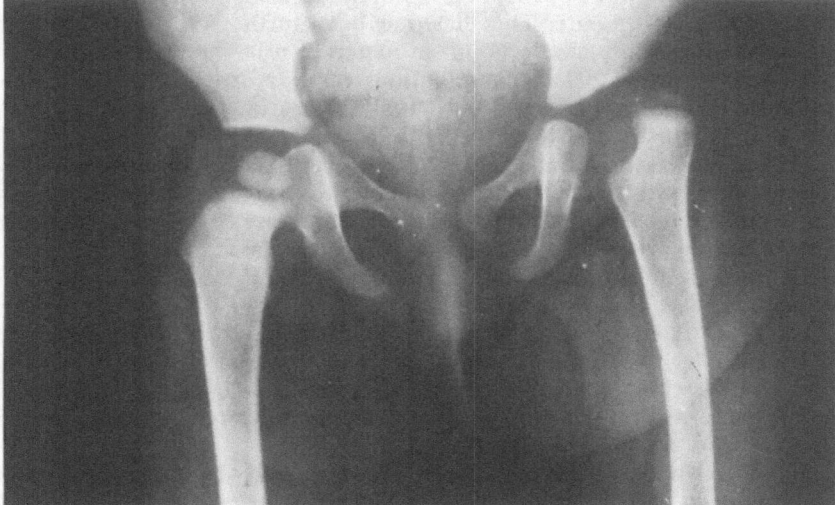

Fig. 1.3. A subluxated hip in a child aged 1 year. With the leg in neutral rotation the head and neck point forwards because of the excessive anteversion

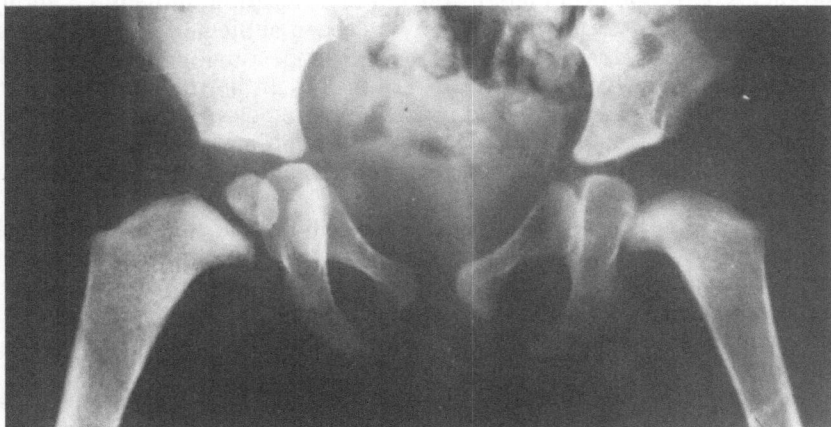

Fig. 1.4. The same hip as in Fig. 1.3, with the leg in full medial rotation

Mechanism of Displacement

Capsular laxity cannot cause displacement; it can only allow it to occur. Some mechanism of displacement is required.

Dennis Browne (1936) described the condition of the compression baby in which the child was crushed in utero in cases of oligohydramnios. He suggested that this was the cause of all typical congenitally dislocated hips and considered that the mechanism of displacement was pressure on the flexed knee forcing the head of the femur out through the back of the acetabulum. He supported this view by showing that the feet of children with dislocated hips were sometimes in calcaneovalgus due to intra-uterine pressure, but were seldom in equinovarus, a deformity which he considered was not due to pressure. This view has been further elaborated by Dunn (1976), who has had an immense amount of experience in the examination of children at birth and in post-mortem examinations of those who have died at birth. He is convinced from what he has seen that all dislocations are caused in this way. There are several difficulties with this theory, however.

Firstly, while there can be no doubt whatever that the compression baby syndrome is a very real entity, it is also certain that babies with this condition look as if they have been subjected to trauma and it comes as a surprise to no-one to find that their hips are dislocated, whereas with a typical congenital dislocation of the hip the baby looks quite normal; in fact the difficulty is to make the diagnosis at all, and this can only be done by a close and careful examination.

Secondly, typical congenital dislocation of the hip is almost eight times as common in girls as it is in boys. This does not definitely rule out the theory, because it may be that compression plus some other factor, such as capsular laxity, is a necessary condition for the milder cases of compression syndrome, but it must cast some doubt upon it.

Thirdly, when the dislocation is unilateral the displacement is four times as commonly on the left side as on the right. Again this may not rule out the hypothesis, because the side affected may be determined by the intrauterine position during parturition (Dunn 1969).

Fourthly, if the dislocation occurs as a result of compression it must be present in utero. This would be supported by dissections which have been carried out post mortem on stillborn infants in which inversion of the limbus has been demonstrated. While this is taken to imply that the hip was dislocated in utero there are certain problems. No child ever died of congenital dislocation of the hip, although children may occasionally die with it. If they had been subjected to sufficient intrauterine trauma to cause death the diagnosis would be obvious and they would not be classified as having typical dislocation of the hip. If they died of some other cause the dislocation might have occurred at birth but the post-mortem examination may not have been undertaken for some hours, by which time rigor mortis would have set in and the changes found would be post mortem and not an indication of intrauterine damage.

The specimen in Fig. 1.5 shows an inverted limbus produced artificially by dislocating the hip in a stillborn infant and then immersing it in formal saline. This had to be done because of the extreme difficulty in obtaining permission to carry out post-mortem examinations within a few hours of death before rigor mortis has set in. All the changes are without doubt post mortem and it can be seen that the limbus is turned in in a very characteristic manner.

The view has been presented that the dislocation occurs superiorly as a result of extension of the hip against the resistance of the flexion contracture present in newborn children.

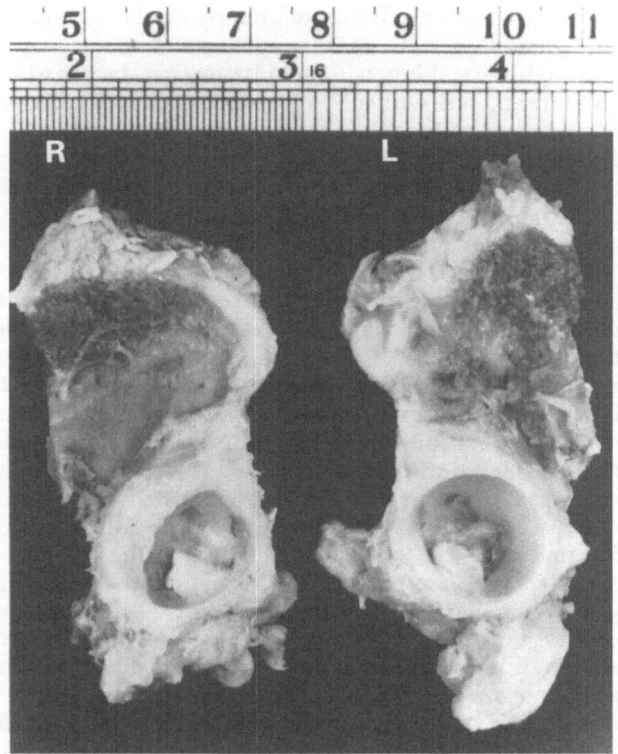

Fig. 1.5. Acetabula of a stillborn child. In the *left* hip the acetabulum is normal but the *right* hip was artificially dislocated and kept in this position for a day or more. The dissected specimen shows the hip limbus inverted in a realistic manner

Mercer (1936) and later O'Malley (1963) suggested that the problem lay in the psoas muscle, which had shortened so that when the hip was forcibly extended the tight psoas acted as a fulcrum about which the head was levered out of the acetabulum. Such a mechanism would force the head of the femur against the posterosuperior part of the acetabulum, and if strong enough would produce a dislocation or subluxation. If the leg were adducted at the same time this might be possible, and this may be the way in which posterior dislocations occur; these behave quite differently from the anterior dislocations more usual in Britain.

The possibility remains that the displacement is initially anterior (Somerville 1953). Such a suggestion is supported by the fact that most of the dislocations and all the subluxations end up in this position and have attained this position obviously by the age of 9 months, and often before. But because the femoral head lies in this position, when the displacement is established there is no certainty that this is the direction in which it occurred; it is very suggestive, however. In such a hip, when it is in full extension, the femoral head lies anterosuperiorly, but in flexion it lies posteriorly. The difficulty in examining the hip in the newborn is that at birth there is a flexion contracture of 45° or more, and with this degree of flexion the position of the femoral head will be either posterior or reduced, depending on the amount of capsular laxity.

Anteversion is the equivalent of lateral rotation of the hip. The arc of rotation of the femoral head in the acetabulum when the hip is in extension is usually about 90°, but whether this arc is predominantly medial or lateral is determined by the angle of anteversion.

Roughly speaking, with no anteversion the arc of rotation will be 45° medial and 45° lateral, but with 45° of anteversion 45° will be subtracted from the lateral rotation and added to the medial rotation, giving an arc of 90° medial rotation and 0° of lateral rotation. This is readily demonstrable in the older child but is obscured by the flexion contracture in the newborn. The rotational arc is quite different with the hip in flexion, when a full normal range in either direction is possible whatever the angle of anteversion.

In a child aged a year or 18 months or more, it can be demonstrated that if there is an increased angle of anteversion (shown by the fact that there is a good deal more medial than lateral rotation in the extended hips) the legs can quite easily be put into the foetal position of full flexion, lateral rotation and some abduction. If such hips are extended fully to lie side by side it can be demonstrated that before this position can be obtained the hips must be medially rotated to the neutral. If the hip is forcibly held in lateral rotation and is not allowed to rotate medially, the head will be forced against the anterior capsule, which if weakened would become stretched and allow displacement. This can also be demonstrated in the stillborn foetal hip if all soft structures are removed or incised to allow full extension and adduction. It is interesting that if all the soft tissues, including the capsule, are excised, leaving only the negative pressure or 'suction' to maintain the femoral head in position the same phenomenon is present with a breaking of the suction seal immediately displacement occurs, indicating that only a very little capsular stretching is necessary to allow subluxation which may rapidly become dislocation. The power of suction is considerable on a straight pull, but the seal is instantly broken on lateral rotation.

It cannot be over-emphasised that any extension, forceful or not, of the hips of a newborn child is potentially dangerous to the hips. Obstetricians and all concerned with parturition should be restrained from holding the child up by the legs and smacking its bottom to stimulate respiration. They should lift the child by the thighs with the hips flexed. They should also be dissuaded from laying the child down flat and extending the hips to measure its length, which is a completely useless exercise. Swaddling with legs extended, practised by many races in one form or another, should be discouraged.

In children with unilateral dislocation of the hip who have grown up it is found (Somerville 1978) that in 20% there is a persistence of anteversion of 45° in the opposite hip, shown by the presence of 90° of medial rotation and 0° lateral rotation. This suggests that the child was born with an excessive degree of anteversion. On one side this led to displacement. On the other side the anteversion was moulded away in 80% of the children but persisted in the other 20%. The inference is that though anteversion is not the cause of displacement, a hip in which there is an excessive degree of anteversion at birth is more at risk than the hip which has a lesser degree (Le Damany 1905).

While the great majority of congenitally dislocated hips in Britain are anterior or anterosuperior, hips are sometimes encountered in which the head lies superior, and much less frequently posterior to the acetabulum. It is difficult to know whether these are stages in a continuing process starting with subluxation and progressing gradually to the most extreme degree of displacement which is posterior (Fig. 1.6), a process that may be halted at any stage, or whether the ultimate displacement occurs all at once with an acute stretching of the capsule and then remains unchanged. It is interesting that posterior dislocation is, with very few exceptions, bilateral and is very rarely seen under the age of 4 years despite its being the most obvious of all the different degrees of displacement, with an obvious waddle and pronounced lordosis.

If it is present all the time why is it missed? If it develops gradually along the lines indicated in the diagram in Fig. 1.6, why is the angle of anteversion very little increased or not even increased at all? It is possible that having reached the posterior position the factors which had been causing an increase of anteversion, which will be described later, will now be reversed and the angle of anteversion will gradually decrease. One can only record the facts, for which there is still no really satisfactory explanation as far as this type of dislocation is concerned.

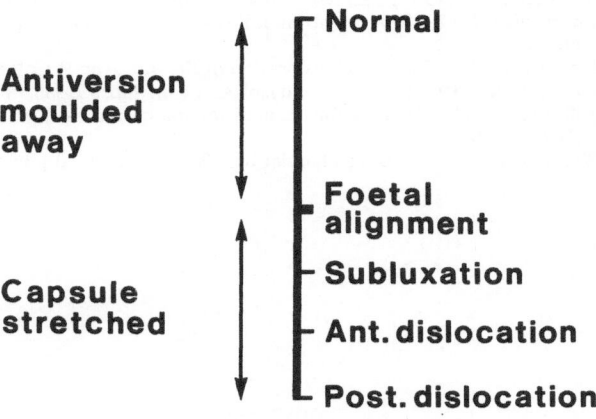

Fig. 1.6. The development of normal and displaced hips shown diagrammatically. All hips must lie between the top and bottom of this scale

The evidence presented here for the possible ways in which displacement occurs must necessarily be inconclusive, because much of it is bound to be conjecture. But a constant review of the material available and the way in which the hip responds to treatment gives a firm impression that the displacement takes place anteriorly due to temporary capsular inadequacy—not just laxity—and that once displacement has become established secondary changes will develop: these will be structural and permanent as a result of the faulty mechanics that have developed.

This monograph is concerned with the nature of these structural changes, the way in which they develop, and the way in which normal growth can be restored by the restoration of normal mechanics.

REFERENCES

Andren L (1960) Acta Radiol (Stockh) 54:123
Andren L (1962) Pelvic instability in newborns. Acta Radiol [Suppl] (Stockh) 212:1
Andren L, Borglin NE (1961) Disturbed urinary excretion pattern of oestrogens in newborns with congenital dislocation of the hip. 1. The excretion of oestrogen during the first few days of life. Acta Endocrinol (Copenh) 37:423
Barlow TG (1966) Congenital dislocation of the hip in the newborn. Proc R Soc Med 59:1103
Browne D (1936) Congenital deformities of mechanical origin. Proc R Soc Med 29:1409
Carter C, Wilkinson JA (1964) Persistent joint laxity in congenital dislocation of the hip. J Bone Joint Surg [Br] 64:40
Dunn PM (1969) Congenital dislocation of the hip. Necropsy studies at birth. Proc R Soc Med 62:1035
Dunn PM (1976) Perinatal observations on the aetiology of congenital dislocation of the hip. Clin Orthop 119:11

Hass J (1948) Congenital dislocation of the hip. Thomas, Springfield

Le Damany P (1905) Une nouvelle théorie pathogénique. Rev Chir 24:175

Le Damany P (1908) Die angeborene Hüftgelenksverrenkung. Z Orthop Chir 21:129

Lloyd-Roberts GC, Swann M (1966) Pitfalls in the management of congenital dislocation of the hip. J Bone Joint Surg [Br] 48:666

Mercer W (1936) Orthopaedic surgery. Arnold, London

O'Malley AG (1963) The influence of flexor and adductor muscles on the hip joint. Clin Orthop 31:73

Salter RB (1970) Text book of disorders and injuries of the musculo-skeletal system. Williams & Wilkins, Baltimore

Somerville EW (1953) Development of congenital dislocation of the hip. J Bone Joint Surg [Br] 35:106

Somerville EW (1959) Paralytic dislocation of the hip. J Bone Joint Surg [Br] 41:279

Somerville EW (1978) A long-term follow-up of congenital dislocation of the hip. J Bone Joint Surg [Br] 60:25

Trevor D (1972) Congenital dislocation of the hip. Ann R Coll Surg Engl 70:213

Weissman SL (1954) Congenital dysplasia of the hip. J Bone Joint Surg [Br] 36:385

Wilkinson JA (1963) Prime factors in the aetiology of congenital dislocation of the hip. J Bone Joint Surg [Br] 45:268

Wynne-Davies R (1970) Acetabular dysplasia and familial joint laxity. J Bone Joint Surg [Br] 52:704

2 Age 0-9 Months

The importance of early diagnosis was first propounded by Putti (1927, 1929). In 1937 Ortolani described a test to enable the diagnosis to be made at the time of birth. In 1962 von Rosen in Malmo and Barlow in Salford reported excellent results of treatment obtained following early diagnosis, with very few failures.

It was unfortunate that all this initial success presented a rather misleading picture to others who tried the same thing. Subsequent experience has shown that neither the problem of early diagnosis nor the problem of early treatment is easy. Both are strewn with difficulties.

EARLY DIAGNOSIS

The two essentials for early diagnosis are organisation and experience. For children born in hospital the problem of organisation is not too difficult. It is not possible for every newborn child to be examined by the orthopaedic surgeon. In most obstetric units the newborn babies are examined by the paediatrician, and it is not too difficult to arrange for an examination of the hips to be included in the routine examination. The difficulty is that all too often this examination is allocated to a resident who, whether senior or junior, will at first have little or no experience in doing the tests and at the end of 6 months will probably be changed for another resident who in turn will be without experience. It is often better for the tests to be performed by a sister, who is less likely to be moved about than a resident, or a general practitioner who regularly visits the hospital, who can gain the necessary experience and have the advantage of continuity. Such a scheme has been reported on very favourably by Moore (1974) in Cork, where the results have shown a great improvement over the previous arrangements.

When the child is born in a small cottage hospital or in the home the difficulty is greater, and it is important that all those concerned with the delivery of children should have instruction in carrying out the tests. It should be the responsibility of the orthopaedic unit covering the area to ensure that this is done, not just once but regularly.

It is now appreciated that the great majority of hips which are unstable at birth will have become stable by the end of the first week of life (Barlow 1966). All hips which are suspect should be seen by an orthopaedic surgeon on about the seventh day after birth. There should be no difficulty in arranging for the child to be seen automatically either at the next orthopaedic out-patient clinic or in the obstetric ward if the child is still in hospital. The examination should be carried out by the surgeon in person and not by a junior, who may have no more experience than the paediatric resident. Teaching of the resident should be carried out with care, remembering that great damage, which is irreversible, can be done by a rough examination.

If the hip is found to be normal no treatment is advised, but the child should be seen again routinely and radiography performed at 6 months and again at 1 year: if the hips are still normal the child can then safely be discharged.

The question of hip roentgenograms being taken at the first examination must be considered. There are some surgeons who believe that this should be done, but if carried to its logical conclusion this would mean x-ray examination of all those hips in which the results of clinical examination are negative. The cost and labour would be very great and the resultant benefit would be minimal. But there is also the problem of making the diagnosis with certainty by means of x-rays. In many unstable hips the head of the femur is sometimes in the joint and sometimes out. If the x-ray picture is taken when the femoral head happens to be in the acetabulum a false-negative will be obtained, so that the value of the x-ray examination will be lost and the false result positively misleading. It seems better to try to improve our clinical skill in making the diagnosis and to use x-rays only at 6 months and 1 year, when there is no doubt that they will be useful.

There is a great temptation for the inexperienced examiner to treat a child with splintage when in doubt, just to be on the safe side, on the basis that it is better to splint too many than too few. At first sight this may seem to be a sensible approach but there are two things to be taken into consideration: Firstly, such a policy will make a nonsense of any statistical survey of the results, because it will be uncertain how many of the hips ever had anything wrong with them, for many would never have needed treatment at all. Secondly, putting the hips of a newborn child into wide abduction is by no means free from complications, and should not be done without good reason.

If it were not for these disadvantages there would be much to be said for adopting a policy of treating all children at birth, at least in those communities where hip dislocation is common.

In some countries it is the practice to treat all unstable hips on the day of birth. In assessing the results of such treatment it should be borne in mind that at least 60% of the hips would have got better without treatment; failure to remember this will produce unjustifiably good results.

In spite of every care it is regrettably the case that a certain number of unstable hips are missed, and that dislocation may occur gradually during the first few months of life. For this reason it is wise to organise some back-up examination some months after birth. This examination can be performed automatically at the time when the routine vaccination and inoculations are done at the age of 4 months.

EXAMINATION

The technique of examination is simple; it requires experience rather than skill. Sometimes simple inspection suggests a difference between the two legs. The thigh may look shorter and as the child kicks freely one hip may be seen to abduct more freely than the other. The creases may be different on the two legs. But inspection alone is often misleading and more often than not the two legs look identical.

The child should be warm, well fed and comfortable; it is impossible to examine an irritable, screaming child. It should be laid on its back on a firm surface and the hips and knees flexed to 90° (Figs. 2.1 and 2.2). The examining hands should hold the thighs with the thumbs on the inner sides and the fingers behind the greater trochanters. In the Ortolani (1937) test the thighs are simply abducted. Normally abduction should be through 90° but sometimes it will be a little less without being abnormal.

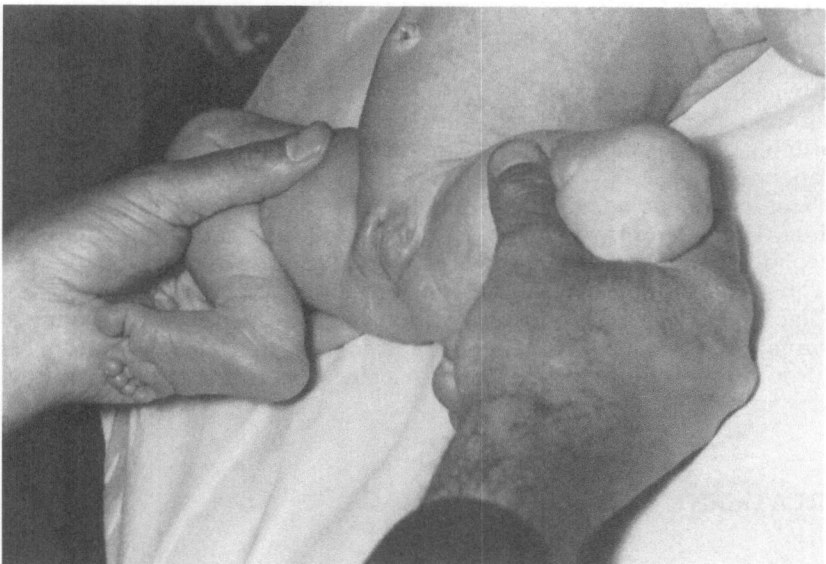

Fig. 2.1. Position of the child and the hands of the examiner during the Ortolani test

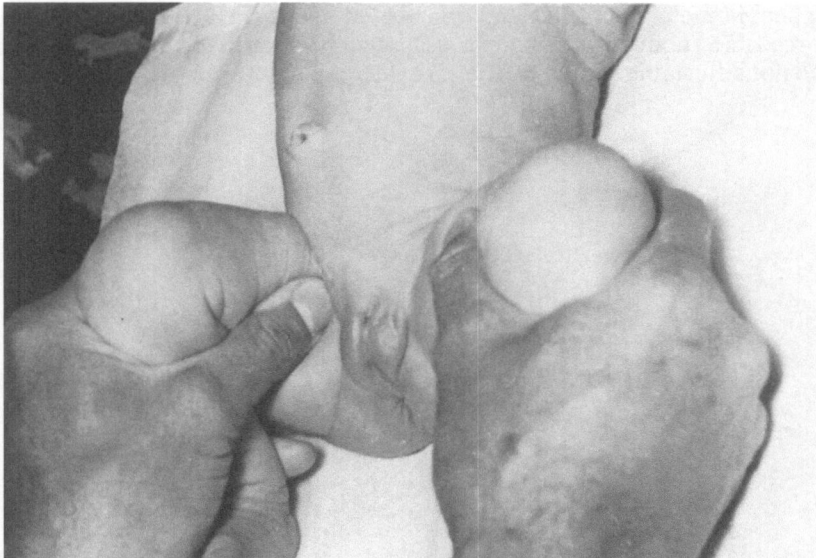

Fig. 2.2. The Barlow test being carried out on the right hip. The examiner's thumb is placed over the femoral head and will displace it backwards and laterally if it is dislocatable

Sometimes the limitation may be more marked, and if when the limit is reached the fingers lift the trochanter forwards there may be a sudden 'clunk' as the head of the femur slips forward over the posterior lip of the acetabulum into the joint. This has been described as a 'click', but there are many clicks in childrens' hips that are of no significance and can be safely ignored. A clunk is very definite; it can be felt, seen, and sometimes even heard.

The Barlow (1962) test is designed to pick out hips with potential instability in which at the time of the examination the head of the femur happens to be in the acetabulum. The limb is held as for the Ortolani test but the thumb is placed more proximally on the inner side of the upper end of the femur. The thigh is first adducted and the tumb gently but firmly pushes the head of the femur laterally. If the hip is unstable displacement will occur and the head will then be reduced by the Ortolani manoeuvre.

This is a valuable test, but it should not be carried out with too much force or too often. Two attempts should be enough, and if displacement has not occurred at the second attempt the result should be considered negative. Too-strenous or too-frequent performance of the test may produce stretching of the capsule and lead to instability which is not apparent at the time. In a hip which was going to develop normally it is possible that this goes on to actual displacement, which may account for a proportion of those hips in which displacement is thought to have developed late after an initially negative examination.

TREATMENT

If the diagnosis is positive some form of splintage will be required, and there are many on the market. All these splints are designed to maintain the hips in a position of abduction. They can be divided into the soft pillow type like the Frejka, the malleable metal splint like the von Rosen splint (Fig. 2.3), and the plastic gutter. Forced fixed abduction is dangerous, as will be described, and no splint which is fixed and not adjustable should be used. In this respect the von Rosen splint is satisfactory

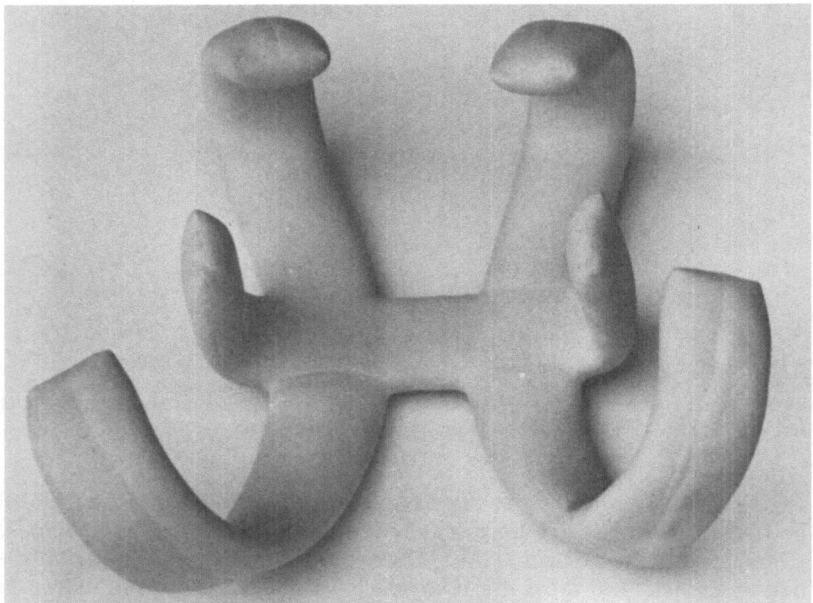

Fig. 2.3. The malleable splint covered in plastic, which was designed by von Rosen

if carefully used, but it must never be applied in such a way as to force the hips into wide abduction.

The shoulder and waist bars are bent up into position before the child is placed on the splint. The hips are then reduced and care is taken to maintain reduction while the child is placed on the splint and the leg bars are bent up around the thighs, but sufficiently loosely to allow the child to kick. At no time must the splint be so tight as to hold the legs in forced abduction. The splint is in fact applied slightly 'inefficiently'.

The mother is given instruction in how to manage the child on the splint. With the child lying supine it is no great problem to wash, dry and powder about three-quarters of the skin surface, and with the child lying prone the splint stands away from the child so that the back can be similarly treated and the splint kept clean and dry. The nappy is worn outside the splint, so that at no time need the splint be removed.

After the child has been placed on the splint no x-ray picture is taken for 1 week, because it can be assumed that the hip was reduced when the splint was applied. It is important to know that the hip has remained reduced at the end of a week when the x-ray picture is taken. If this is satisfactory the child is kept on the splint for 3 months without further x-ray or other examinations. It is difficult to believe that anything but harm can come from the practice of removing the child at intervals from the splint to see whether the hip has become stable in the meantime.

At the end of 3 months the child is removed from the splint and is allowed to kick freely for 1 month. By the end of this time the child will have regained adduction, so that an x-ray picture can be taken with the legs together. It is only with the legs in this position that true reduction can be claimed.

The child is allowed to remain free without any restrictions and reviewed again at the end of a further 6 months, with an x-ray picture again taken with the legs together. This is repeated at the end of 2 years, and all being well the child can then be safely discharged.

Complications

As already mentioned, the treatment of this condition is fraught with dangers; the complications are serious and they are almost all iatrogenic.

TIGHTNESS OF THE ADDUCTOR MUSCLES

Tightness of the adductor muscles leads to the most serious complications. If the adductors are very tight it is unlikely that harm will be done, because it will be difficult or impossible to put the child onto the splint without carrying out an adductor tenotomy. The danger arises when the adductors are only slightly tight; sometimes this may be so slight that at the time of treatment it was not recognised. In these circumstances any forced abduction will put pressure on the femoral head, squeezing blood out of the epiphysial vessels and producing ischaemia. That this has happened may not become apparent for many months, until it becomes obvious that the development of the ossific nucleus has been delayed; and when it does appear it will often be multinucleated (Fig. 2.4). As the head grows the nuclei will fuse but the head will often develop with some persistent deformity, leading to deformity of the acetabulum and inevitable arthritis in later life (Fig. 2.5). It seems that there is a greater likelihood of this deformity developing following ischaemia in the newborn than when it develops following treatment of the rather older child.

A more serious deformity resulting from pressure on the femoral head develops

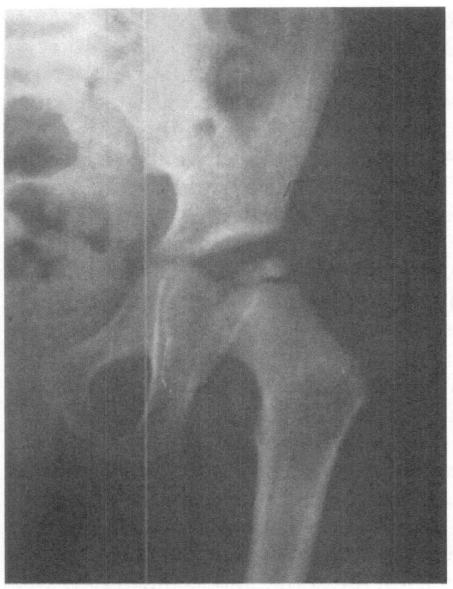

Fig. 2.4. Multinucleated development of the ossific nucleus following damage to the blood supply during treatment undertaken at birth

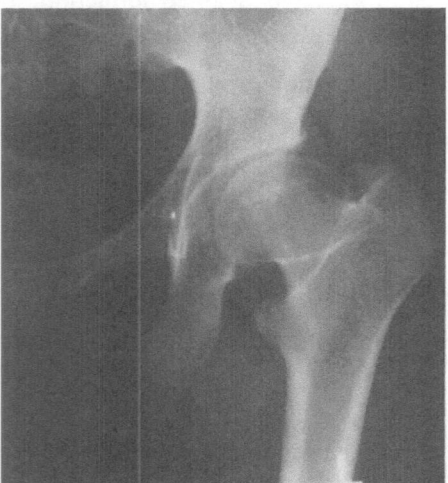

Fig. 2.5. The same hip as in Fig. 2.4 seen 15 years later. There has been damage to the growth plate, leaving a short neck, and the head is mushroomed causing dysplasia of the acetabulum

when damage is done to the growth plate (Fig. 2.6). Such damage is irreversible and largely uncorrectable. That this damage has been done will not usually become apparent for a year or 18 months, and when the damage has been of lesser severity it may not be noticed for several years (Fig. 2.7), and sometimes not until adolescence when the patient is seen because of a limp.

THE UNREDUCED HIP

Children are sometimes referred who have been placed on the splint without the hip having been reduced or have been placed on the splint with the hip reduced but in whom displacement has subsequently developed so that the hip has been splinted in

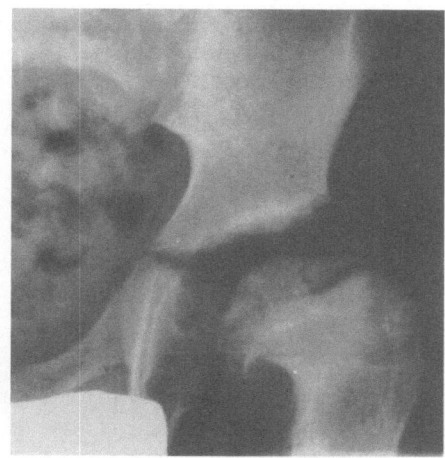

Fig. 2.6. Hip treated 1 week after birth for displacement. The hip was abducted in the frog position for 3 months. Severe damage has been done to the growth plate and to the blood supply of the ossific nucleus. Such changes are irreversible

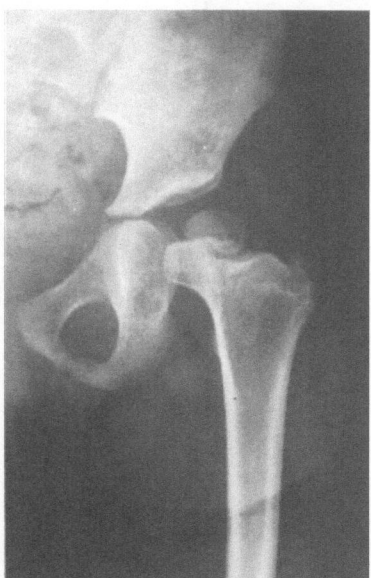

Fig. 2.7. Similar case to the one shown in Fig. 2.6, but the damage is much less severe. While the growth plate has been damaged it appears that the ossific nucleus has been spared. This is the sort of deformity which may pass undetected for many years

the frog position for 3 months (Fig. 2.8) with the hip still dislocated. In this position the head of the femur will lie behind the acetabulum as seen in the model (Fig. 2.9), with the posterior aspect of the head against the back of the acetabulum. This continual pressure will gradually force the upper end of the femur into an extreme degree of anteversion (Fig. 2.10). The treatment of this difficult problem will be described later (p. 142).

REDISPLACEMENT

It is very uncommon for redislocation to occur following treatment shortly after birth. In the past 20 years in Oxford it has only happened on one occasion. By the age of 4 months the child will have reached the age when closed reduction will have become dangerous and operative reduction is unsatisfactory and has nothing to offer over treatment 6 months later. It is probably wiser to withhold treatment until the child is 9 months or a year old rather than reapplying the splint.

Some degree of subluxation seen at the 1-year follow-up is not very uncommon

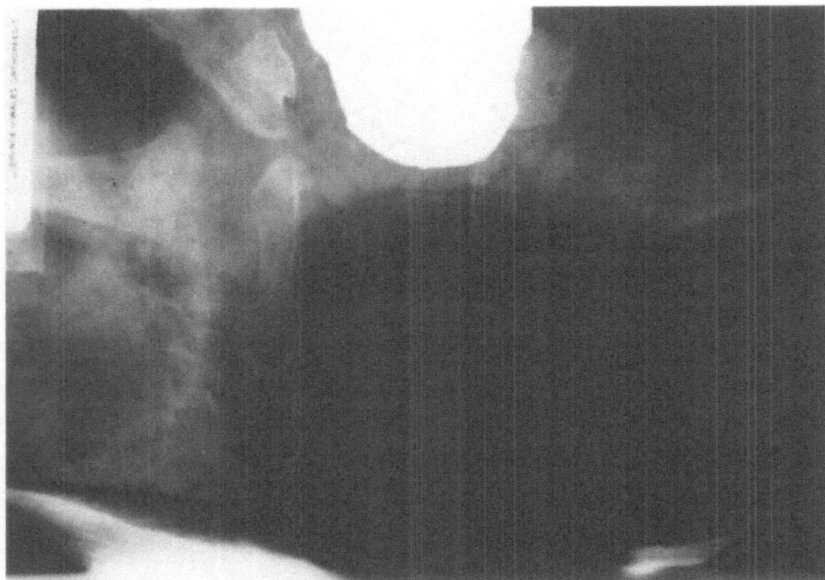

Fig. 2.8. Following early diagnosis the hips were splinted in the frog position for 3 months. When the splint was removed the radiograph showed that the right hip had never been reduced. The left hip had always been normal

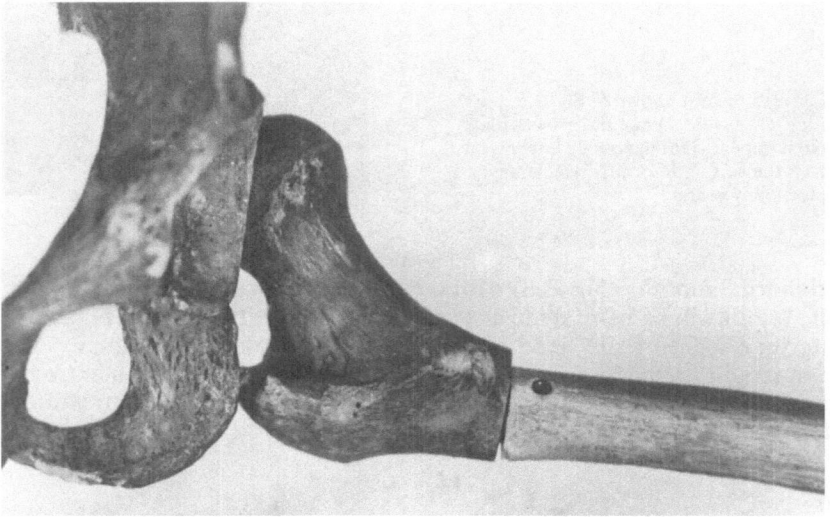

Fig. 2.9. The model demonstrates the position of the head as seen in the radiograph in Fig. 2.8. The posterior aspect of the head is against the posterior aspect of the acetabulum. There is continuous pressure forcing the neck of the femur increasingly into anteversion

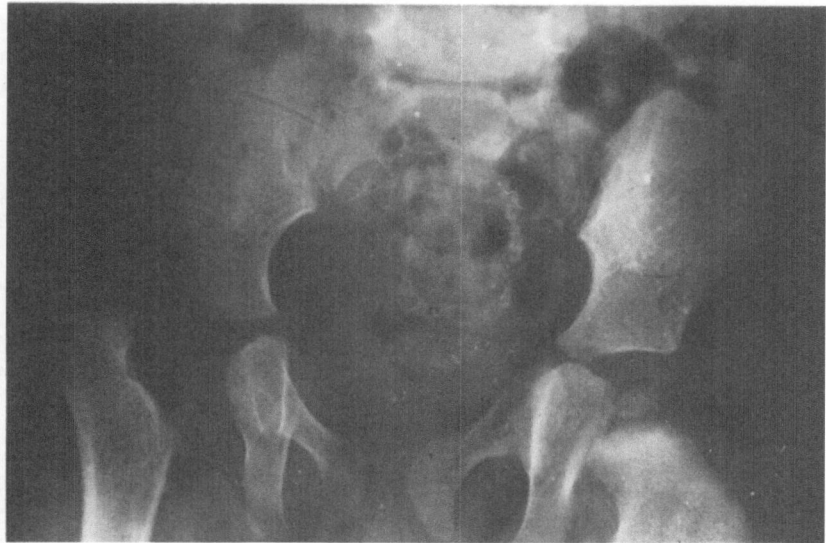

Fig. 2.10. The same hip as seen in Fig. 2.8. The grossly excessive anteversion is clearly seen 18 months later

(Fig. 2.11). It should be ignored and the child allowed to continue to lead a normal life. In the great majority by 2 or 2½ years of age the hips will have developed normally (Fig. 2.12). Very occasionally it will become apparent that spontaneous resolution is not occurring (Fig. 2.13), but if this is the case the hips will develop

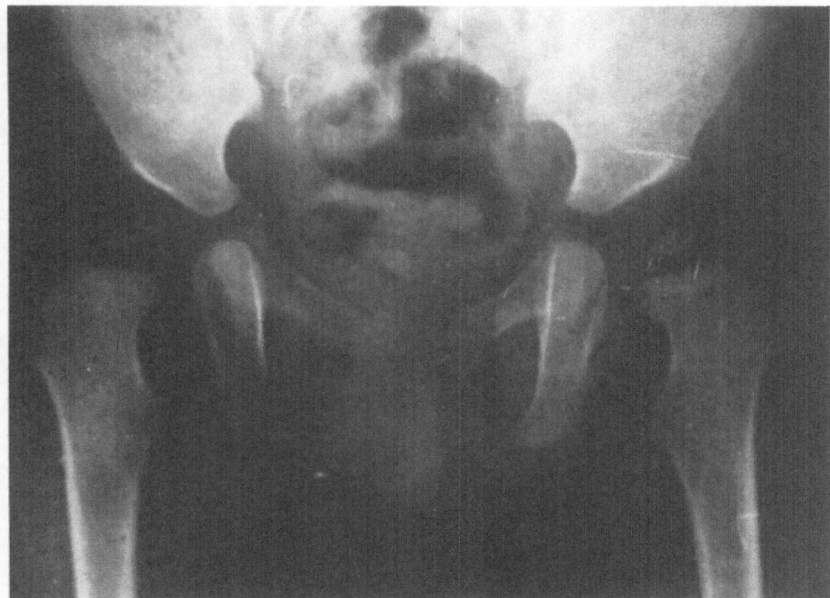

Fig. 2.11. When the splint is first removed it is not uncommon to see the degree of displacement shown here. It rarely causes trouble and needs no special treatment

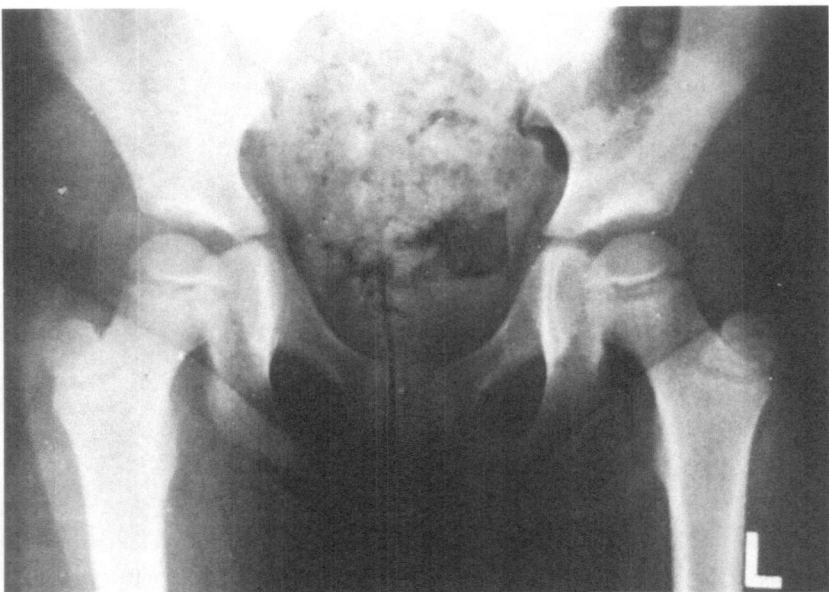

Fig. 2.12. The same hips seen 5 years later. Both have developed normally without treatment

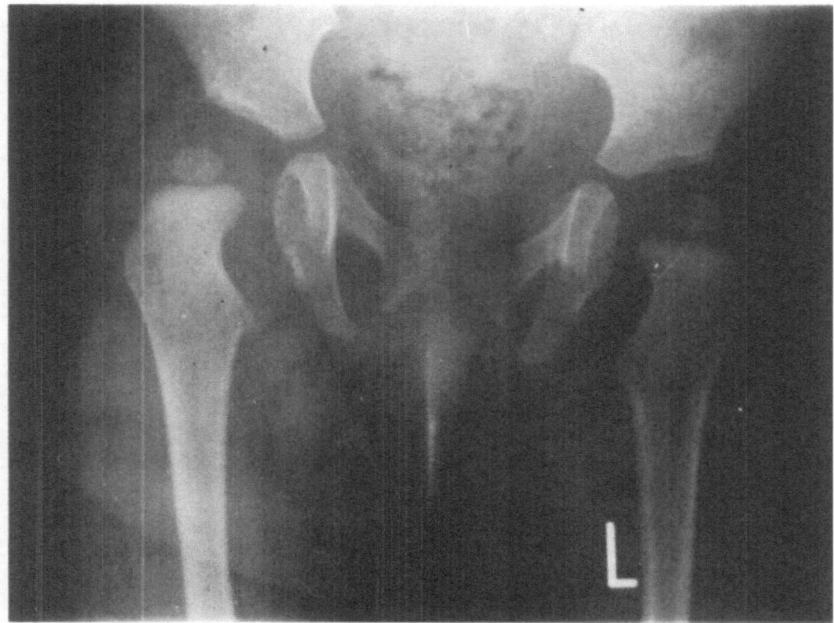

Fig. 2.13. Very occasionally the displacement may persist, as is seen here 2 years after birth. It can easily be corrected by the restoration of normal anteversion by means of a high femoral osteotomy

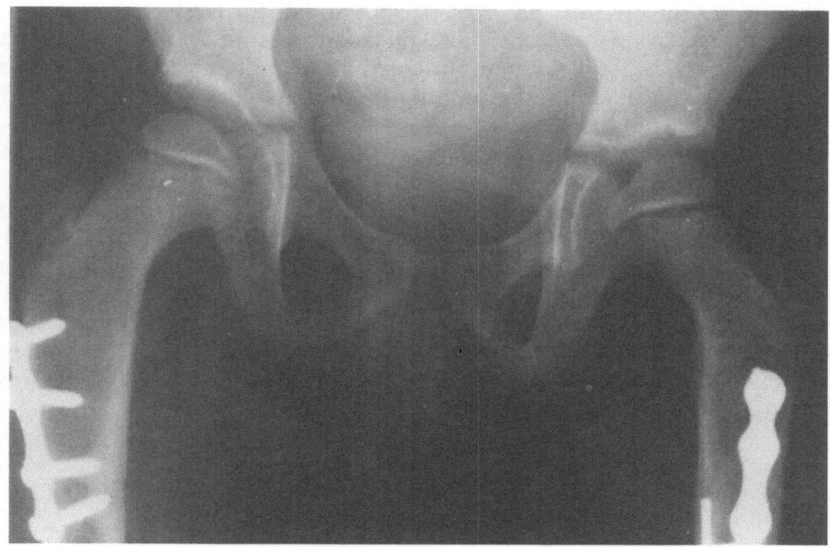

Fig. 2.14. Four years later it can be seen that both the hips shown in Fig. 2.13 are developing well

normally after a suitable high femoral osteotomy (Fig. 2.14). The cause of this failure of spontaneous resolution is probably a persistence of an excessive degree of anteversion.

If at any time during the course of early treatment there is difficulty in maintaining reduction without the use of force it is better to discard all splintage and leave the child to move freely until the age of 9 months or 1 year and then restart treatment, even though at this age treatment will involve operation. There is as yet no certain evidence that early open reduction by the method described by Ludloff (1913) or any other method has a better record than delaying operation until the child is older.

RESULTS OF EARLY DIAGNOSIS AND TREATMENT

Because of the very great difficulty of following up all children who have been examined at birth in a particular unit in sufficient numbers to be of significance and because of the uncertainty as to how many hips initially treated would have undergone spontaneous resolution without treatment for the reasons already mentioned, it is difficult to obtain any reliable statistics. Without such statistics it cannot be said for certain just how valuable this procedure is.

For this reason doubts have been expressed (Wilkinson 1972) as to whether it is worthwhile carrying out these examinations at all and, in view of the risks involved, whether early treatment is justifiable. In our opinion treatment is safe provided it is carried out with care by those who are fully aware of the dangers. But this still leaves the problem of not knowing whether enough positive diagnoses are made to justify it.

We have attempted to make an assessment of this in Oxford, where since 1957 all children born in the Radcliffe Infirmary, The Churchill Hospital, and the John Radcliffe Hospital (opened in 1972) have been examined at birth. The total number of live births during this time was 82 380, and as far as is known all these children were examined. Any in whom the results of hip examination were doubtful were not treated even with double nappies but were re-examined with x-rays at 6 months and again at 1 year. All children attending the welfare clinics for their inoculations at 4 months were again examined.

It is known that in the 20 years from 1957 to 1977, of the 82 380 children examined 31 were subsequently diagnosed in Oxford or in the peripheral hospitals as having dislocated hips. Assuming that the incidence of displacement in Oxford is the same as for the rest of the country, i.e., 1.5 per 1000 live births, it could have been expected that there would have been 126 children with congenital dislocation of the hip. According to the statistics of the Community Medical Service it would be expected that 5%–10% of children would have moved from the area within 2 years of birth, during which time the diagnosis should have been made. From this it can be calculated that rather more than 80 children of the 126 possibles were saved from developing established dislocations.

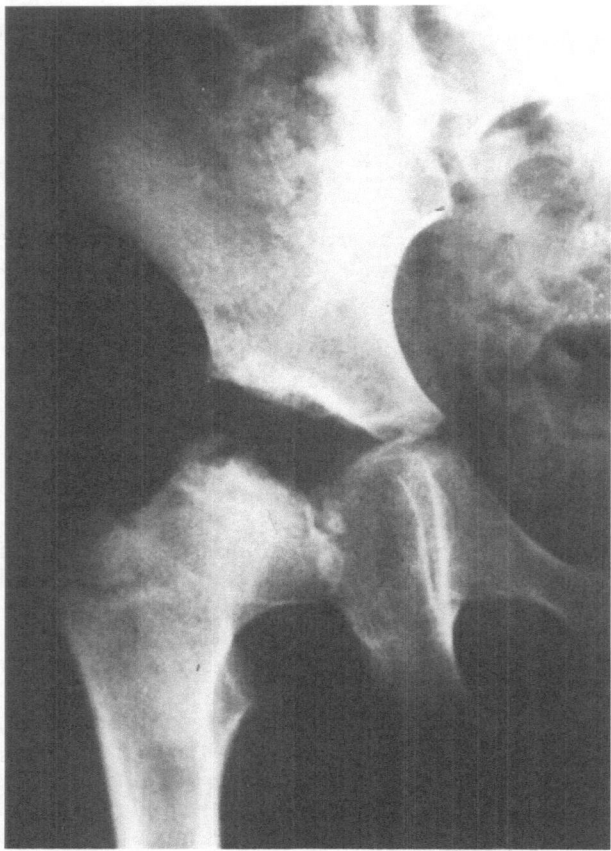

Fig. 2.15. This hip was initially treated when the child was 4 months of age. The hips were put in plaster with more than 90° of flexion and only 45° of abduction. Severe damage was done to the ossific nucleus, which after 7 years is still showing little evidence of recovery although the hip is well reduced

RESULTS OF LATER TREATMENT

Early treatment can be considered as being that given in the first month of life. After that, with every week that passes, the risk of producing damage to the growth plate increases (Fig. 2.15), and unless reduction is very easy it is better to postpone treatment until the age of 9 months or 1 year and then to operate. Alternatively, up to 9 months an apparatus such as the Pavlic sling, which does not seem to do any harm, may be tried. It has proved effective in those hips where there is a moderate degree of instability and displacement, but in our experience so far it has not been so useful in more severe cases. It is a relatively simple webbing harness (Fig. 2.16) which is adjusted so that the child can only extend the hips in abduction but is otherwise able to kick freely. The appliance is worn for about 9 months until it becomes clear whether or not the treatment is going to be effective. It cannot be over-emphasised that rigid fixation in wide abduction, particularly in plaster, must never be used in this age group. The hip shown in Fig. 2.15 was treated at age of 4 months in plaster in 100° flexion and 45° abduction. The child is now aged 7 years, and but for the vascular damage would have had a good result.

Figure 2.17 shows the hip of a child aged 4 months, with a minor degree of displacement. Simple splinting failed to reduce it and an arthrogram shows that the cause of the trouble is a large inverted limbus (Fig. 2.18). Any attempt to persevere with conservative treatment would have caused irreversible damage, but excision of the limbus and rotation osteotomy have produced a good reduction (Fig. 2.19).

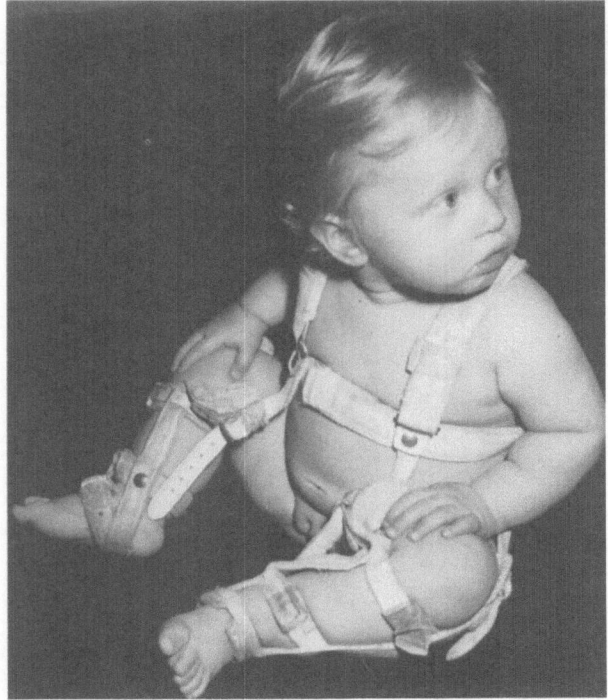

Fig. 2.16. A Pavlic sling worn by an infant

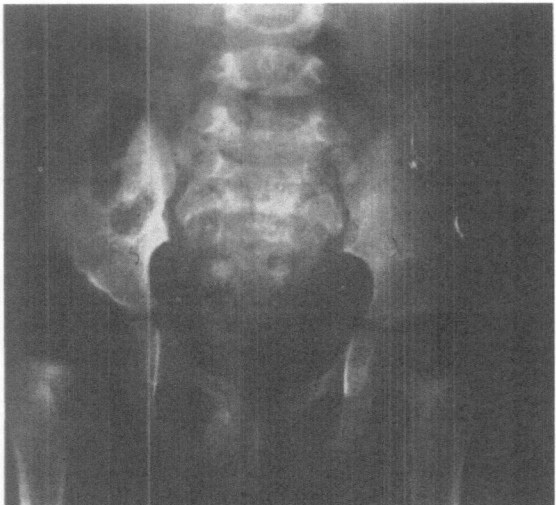

Fig. 2.17. Minor degree of displacement of the left hip in a child aged 4 months. Reduction was not possible

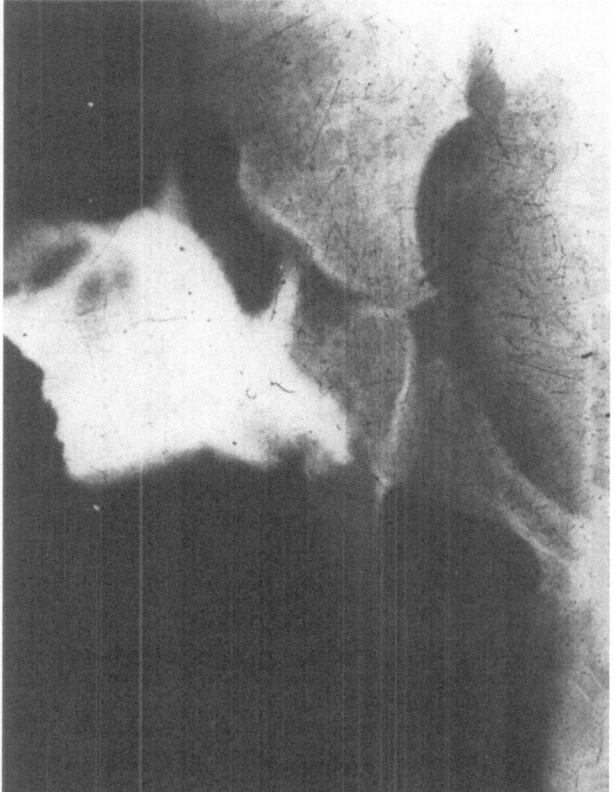

Fig. 2.18. An arthrogam shows that the obstruction in the hip shown in Fig. 2.18 is due to a very large limbus

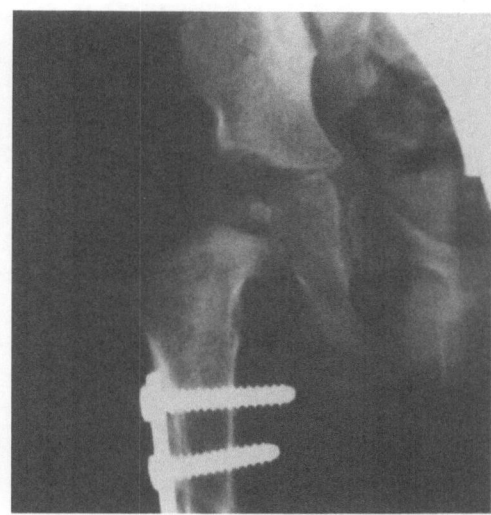

Fig. 2.19. After removal of the limbus it was possible to obtain a good reduction in the hip shown in Fig. 2.18

Although the result here was satisfactory, rotation osteotomy on bones so small is hazardous and it would have been wiser to wait until the child was 9 months or a year old, when surgery would have been safer and the result should have been as good.

REFERENCES

Barlow TG (1962) Early diagnosis and treatment of congenital dislocation of the hip. J Bone Joint Surg [Br] 44:292

Barlow TG (1966) Congenital dislocation of the hip in the new born. Proc R Soc Med 59:1103

Ludloff K (1913) The open reduction of the congenital hip dislocation by an anterior incision. Am J Orthop Surg 10:438

Mau H, Döor WM, Henkel L, Lutsche J (1971) Open reduction of congenital dislocation of the hip by Ludloff's method. J Bone Joint Surg [Am] 53:1281

Mitchell GP (1972) Problems in the early diagnosis and management in congenital dislocation of the hip. J Bone Joint Surg [Br] 54:4

Moore FH (1974) Screening of congenital dislocation of the hip. J Irish Med Assoc 67/4:104

Ortolani M (1937) Un segno poco noto e sua importnaza per la diagnosi precoce di prelussazione congenitala dell'anca. Pediatria 45:129

Putti V (1927) Diagnosi precoce tratament della dussazione congenita dell'anca. Chir Organi Mov 13:529

Putti V (1929) Early treatment of congenital dislocation of the hip. J Bone Joint Surg 11:798

Rosen S von (1962) Diagnosis and treatment of congenital dislocation of the hip in the newborn. J Bone Joint Surg [Br] 44:538

Rosen S von (1968) Further experience with congenital dislocation of the hip in the newborn. J Bone Joint Surg [Br] 50:538.

Salter RB (1970) Text book of disorders and injuries of the musculo-skeletal system. Williams & Wilkins, Baltimore

Trevor D (1972) Congenital dislocation of the hip. Ann R Coll Surg Engl 50:213

Wilkinson JA (1972) A post-natal survey of congenital displacement of the hip. J Bone Joint Surg [Br] 54:40

3 The Secondary Changes

If the golden opportunity for early diagnosis and treatment has been missed and displacement of the head of the femur persists, whether small or great, secondary structural changes will develop, which can become permanent as the likelihood that damage will be irreversible increases with continuing duration of displacement.

Initially, displacement may be so small as to amount to no more than an eccentricity of movement of the head of the femur within the acetabulum. Even this will, with time, lead to a progressive deterioration of the joint, so that there will be some acetabular dysplasia which will be secondary. But more severe degrees of displacement may be present from the start, which will lead to greater changes.

The changes, all of which are secondary to the displacement, are to be found in:—

    1) The ossification
    2) The soft tissues
    3) The acetabulum
    4) The upper end of the femur.

OSSIFICATION

There is delay in the ossification of the whole joint. This will be shown by delay in appearance and under-development of the ossific nucleus in the head of the femur, and an apparent sloping of the acetabular roof. The retarded ossification, together with a minor degree of displacement, can give rise to a most misleading radiograph if it is not correctly interpreted.

The radiograph of the hip of a 17-month-old child (Fig. 3.1) presents at first sight the appearance of an acetabulum with a defective sloping roof with displacement of the femoral head. It is this appearance which has for so long led to a misunderstanding of the nature of this condition. Discussion has ranged round the acetabular 'index', which is the angle between the horizontal and the supposed roof of the acetabulum when all that is being measured is the angle between the horizontal and the visible ossification of the ilium, which, of course, has nothing to do with the shape or size of the acetabulum but only with the degree of ossification.

At this age the hip joint cannot be seen on a plain radiograph, because it is composed entirely of cartilage on both the femoral and pelvic sides of the joint. Nothing can be seen but the centres of ossification. That in the head of the femur is obviously small because ossification has been retarded by the instability of the joint and the eccentricity of movement of the femoral head in the acetabulum.

If these factors cause delay in ossification on the femoral side of the joint it is only to be expected that they will cause the same delay on the acetabular side, as shown by deficient ossification in the ilium giving the appearance of a defective acetabular roof. This can be confirmed by arthrography. Figure 3.2 shows the same hip after the

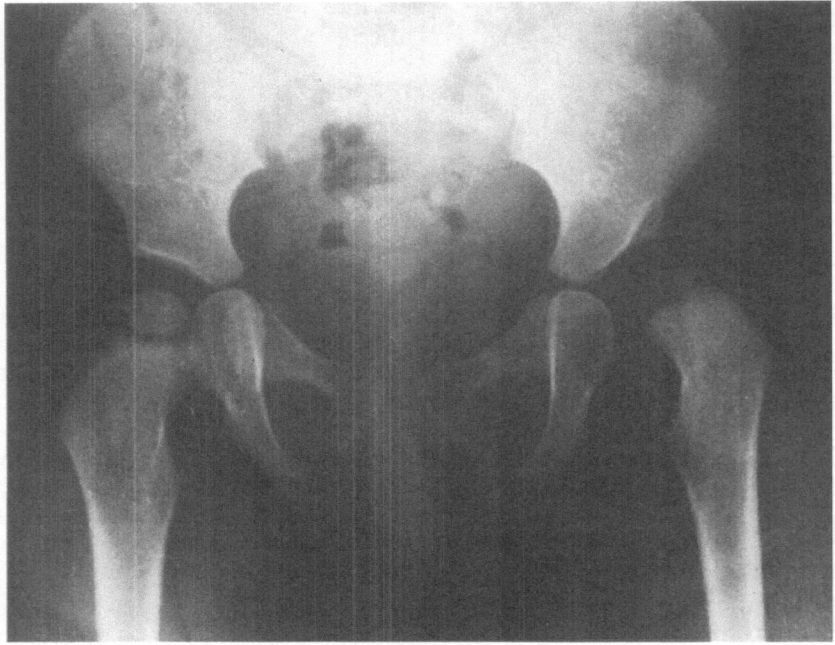

Fig. 3.1. Subluxation of the hip in a child aged 17 months. Retarded ossification on both sides of the joint gives the illusion of a defective acetabulum

injection of a radio-opaque fluid which outlines the true joint. It shows that the shape of the cartilaginous acetabular roof is quite normal and that the femoral head fits it accurately. This is a normal hip. The only abnormality is the capsular laxity.

While instability is one cause for the delay in ossification in the capital ossific nucleus there is a further reason for its small size in some cases: the blood supply is from two leashes of vessels. The larger lies posterolaterally and supplies the anterolateral part of the femoral ossific nucleus. The second leash lies postero-medially and supplies the posteromedial part (Trueta 1957). There is little if any anastomosis between these vessels, so that if one leash is damaged one part of the nucleus will become ischaemic if it is already formed, as in Perthes' disease (Fig. 8.1) where it is the lateral leash which is most commonly affected. If the nucleus has not already appeared, as in the newborn or very young child, its appearance will be much delayed.

This phenomenon is not infrequently seen in congenital dislocation of the hip but it is the medial side of the nucleus which is affected. The reason is clearly seen in the model (Figs 3.3 and 3.4), where it can be seen that in the dislocated position it is the posteromedial part of the head of the femur which is in contact with the pelvis and will knock against the side of the pelvis in movement, and this will endanger the patency of the posteromedial leash of vessels which enter the bone at this point. If it is damaged, in part or in whole, the development of the posteromedial part of the nucleus will be impaired or delayed.

In Fig. 3.5 the lateral part of the ossific nucleus is well formed but the medial part is only just appearing. Two years later it is better defined (Fig. 3.6), and finally it becomes competely incorporated (Fig. 3.7). Figure 3.8 shows the appearance in

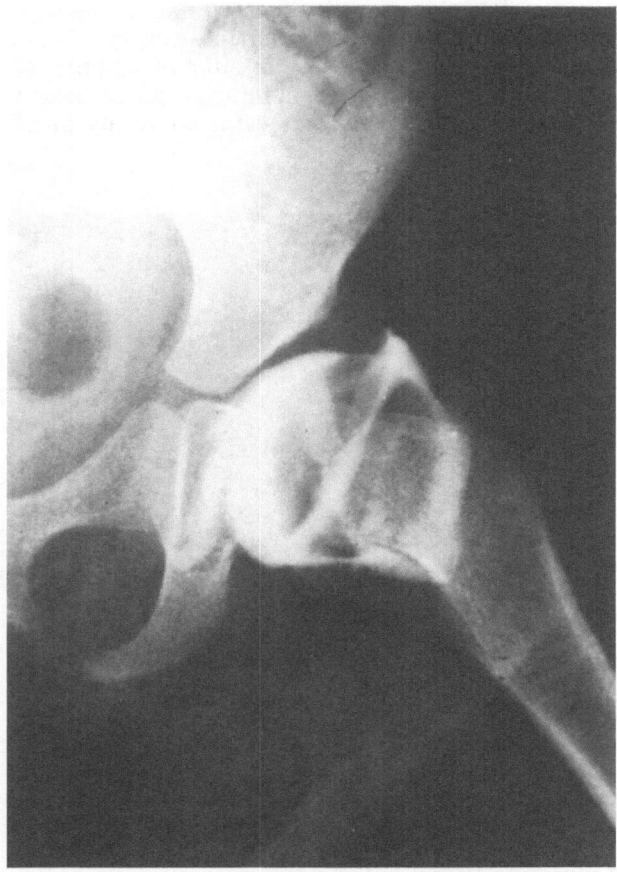

Fig. 3.2. An arthrogram of the same hip as is shown in Fig. 3.1 shows that the acetabular shape is normal, as is the femoral head, which fits it well. Neither could be seen in the straight radiograph because they are composed of cartilage

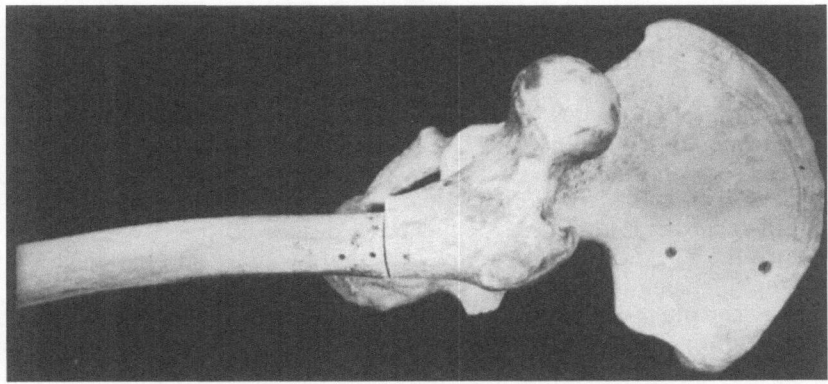

Fig. 3.3. Model showing the position of the femoral head in relation to the pelvis in typical anterior dislocation when the hip is in extension

another child, in whom it appears that the medial side of the femoral head was severely damaged before treatment. Ten years later (Fig. 3.9), it is clear that the blood supply has been restored to the medial part of the nucleus, which has undergone normal ossification even though some damage has been done to the medial part of the growth plate, causing a varus deformity which will persist.

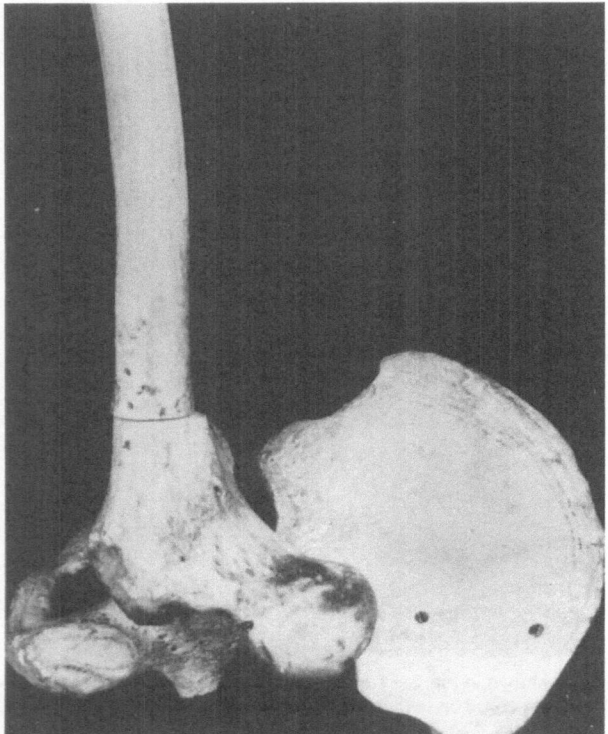

Fig. 3.4. Model showing the position of the femoral head when the hip is in flexion

SOFT TISSUES

The changes in the soft tissues are purely adaptive. Some are adaptively shortened and some are stretched, while others are simply distorted. But because the changes can be so simply explained it does not mean that they are not of importance—just the reverse is the case. It is probable that the soft tissue changes are the most important of all the changes found in the congenitally dislocated hip.

It is the soft tissues alone which maintain two joint surfaces in contact. The shape of the opposing joint surfaces has little effect on stability in any joint, and in some none. The hip is one of the more stable joints, but even this would fall apart if it were not held together by the soft tissues. But by far the most important function is that they are responsible for the type of movement which takes place in the joint. It is the soft tissues which ensure the maintenance of a concentric type of movement and it is a failure of the soft tissues which permits an eccentric type of movement to develop.

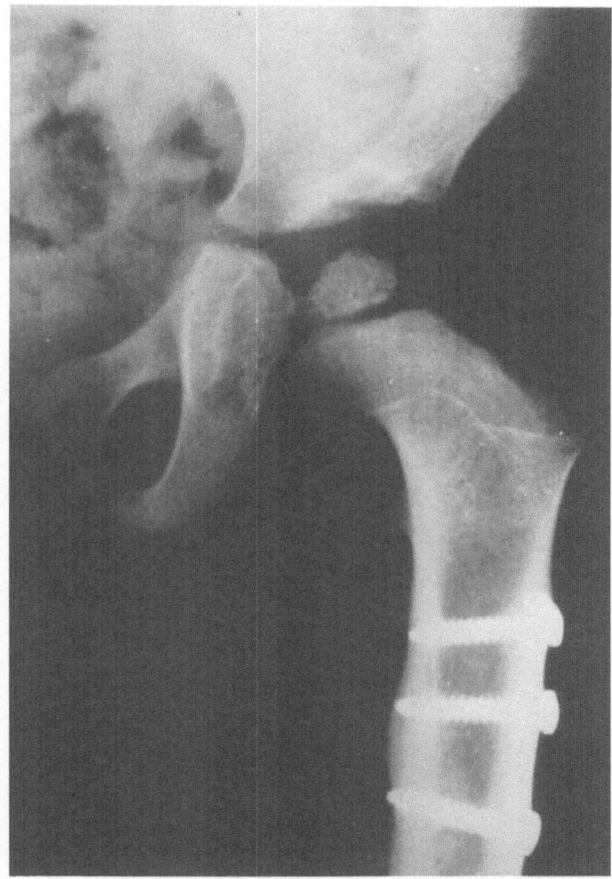

Fig. 3.5. Hip after treatment, showing small medial nucleus. Note: Harris's growth line indicates how the upper end of the femur grows

When a hip is dislocated the soft tissues become adapted to the dislocated position. If the hip is reduced and immediately left free the soft tissues will redislocate it. It is only when the soft tissues have readapted to the reduced position that stable reduction is established, and the soft tissues will then be holding the head of the femur in the acetabulum.

Such readaptation occurs very quickly in the newborn but with increasing difficulty as time passes. It is this difficulty of adaptation which makes the treatment of the older congenitally dislocated hip so difficult and the result so unreliable, rather than the actual deformity which occurs in the bone, though this also plays a part when it becomes established.

DEFORMITY OF THE ACETABULUM

Deformity of the acetabulum depends on the degree of displacement and even more on the type of movement which the displacement, and the soft tissue adaptation to it,

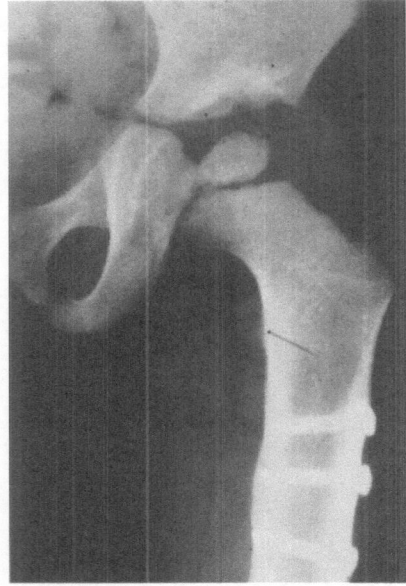

Fig. 3.6. Same hip as in Fig. 3.5, two years later. The medial nucleus is now quite large

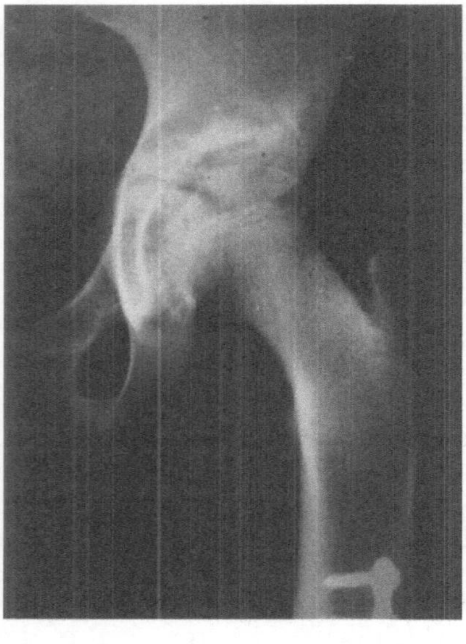

Fig. 3.7. Same hip as in Figs. 3.5 and 3.6, shown 20 years later than in Fig. 3.6. The medial nucleus has now become completely incorporated with the larger lateral nucleus

allows. In the normal hip with concentric movement not only is the head of the femur the centre of movement but the centre of the head of the femur is the centre of movement, so that it simply rotates and does not move about. In subluxation the head of the femur, which is in the acetabulum, is the centre of movement but the centre of the head is not, because there is laxity of the soft tissues allowing the head to slip about in the acetabulum. This is eccentric movement. When the head of the femur is moving in an eccentric manner it will gradually mould the lip of the

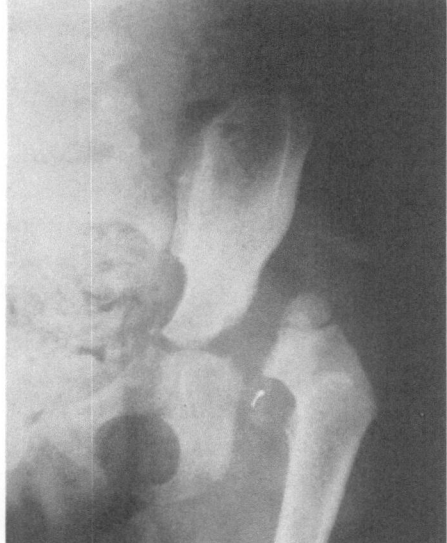

Fig. 3.8. An untreated dislocation in a child aged 2 years, showing damage which has been done to the posteromedial aspect of the head by pressure against the pelvis

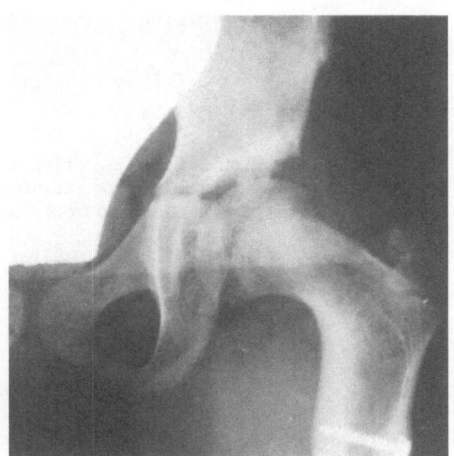

Fig. 3.9. The same hip as in Fig. 3.8, showing that the posteromedial part of the nucleus developed following treatment and became incorporated into the anterolateral portion but that damage had been done to the medial part of the growth plate leading to a varus deformity

acetabulum outwards, the anterosuperior part of the lip being chiefly affected because this is the direction of subluxation.

In dislocation the femoral head is no longer the centre of movement, and as shown in the models (Figs. 3.3 and 3.4) the centre of movement is somewhere in the intertrochanteric region, perhaps closely related to the psoas, on which the femur may well swing. With every movement the head of the femur grinds against the side of the pelvis (Fig. 1.2) and will do most damage to the most prominent part, which will be the lip of the acetabulum posteriorly and superiorly. The lip of the acetabulum or limbus is fibrocartilaginous, soft and malleable, and under repeated pressure it becomes deformed and turned into the joint (Fig. 1.5). Figure 3.10 shows the different degrees of inversion which may be encountered.

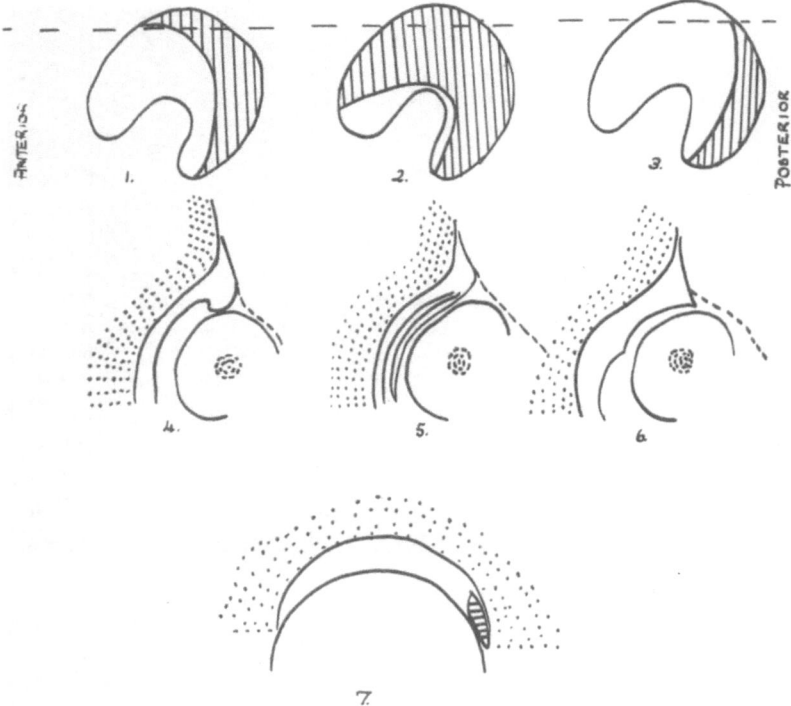

Fig. 3.10. Parts 1, 2, and 3 show diagrammatically the different sizes of the limbus which may be encountered, and parts 4, 5, and 6 show the different arthrographic appearance of each. Part 7 shows how the inverted limbus prevents the head from entering the acetabulum fully

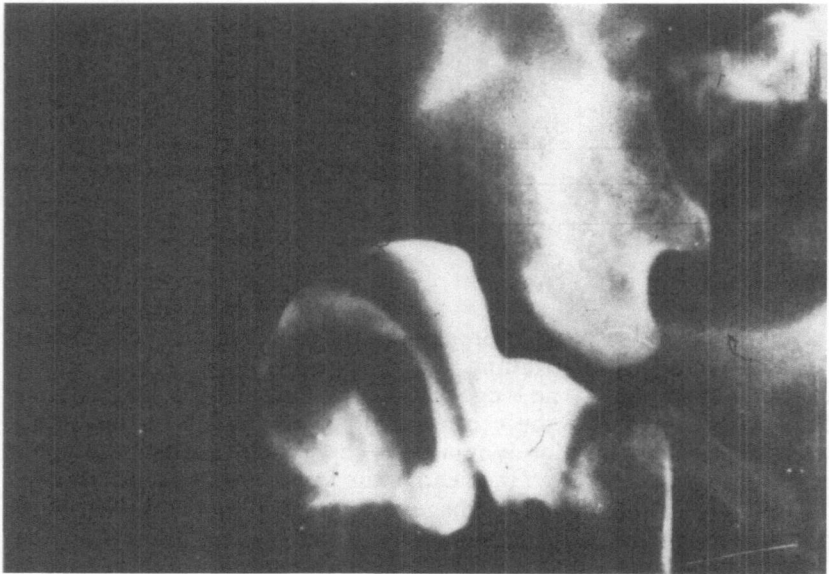

Fig. 3.11. An arthrogram of a dislocated hip in a child aged 1 week. The femoral head is out of the joint but the limbus is not deformed

The limbus is not turned into the joint in a newborn child with a dislocated hip. The arthrogram in Fig. 3.11 shows the head out of the joint, but the limbus is unde-formed. This was a bilateral dislocation and the radiographically visible changes were the same on both sides. Because of the extreme instability it was difficult to maintain reduction and it was considered wiser to postpone treatment until the child was 1 year old. After kicking freely for 10 months the child was readmitted and a further arthrogram showed that the limbus was now turned into the joint in a manner typical of a dislocation (Fig. 3.12).

It is the active kicking of the child which causes the deformity of the limbus. In those cases where the dislocation is associated with some form of paralysis, so that active kicking is nil or restricted, the limbus is rarely deformed at all.

It is interesting that while the eversion of the limbus in subluxation takes place slowly—it may take 2 or 2½ years before it reaches a degree of significance—the inversion of the limbus takes place rapidly and may be established within a few months. Figure 2.18 shows the inverted limbus as seen in an arthrogram at the age of 4 months.

The greater the displacement the less damage is done to the acetabulum, so that in some cases of posterior dislocation in which there is very extensive capsular laxity and the femoral head is far removed from the acetabulum (Fig. 3.13), the degree of grinding against the side of the pelvis is minimal; in such cases little damage, and in some cases no damage, will be done and the limbus will remain undeformed. At the other end of the scale, when the displacement is less (Fig. 3.14) and the head may be lodged on the lip of the acetabulum, maximal damage will be done to it.

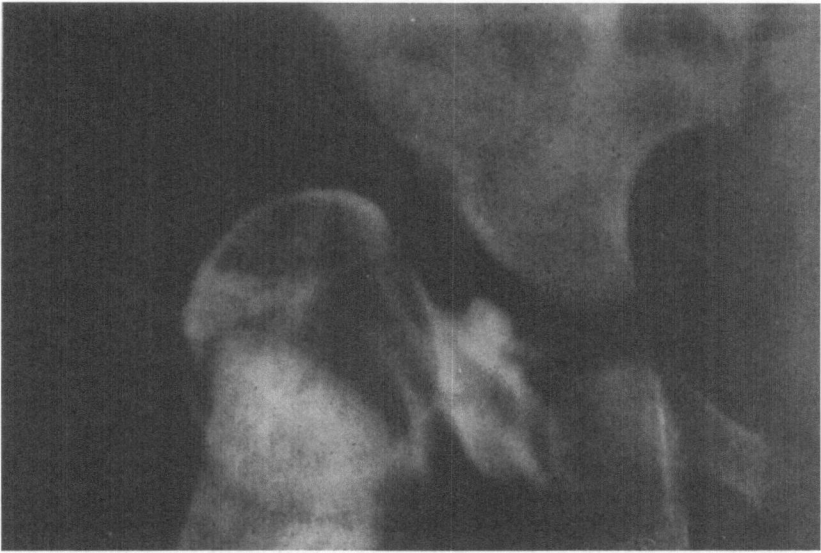

Fig. 3.12. An arthrogram of the same hip as in Fig. 3.11, one year later; the hip has not been treated so that the child has been kicking freely. The limbus is now typically inverted

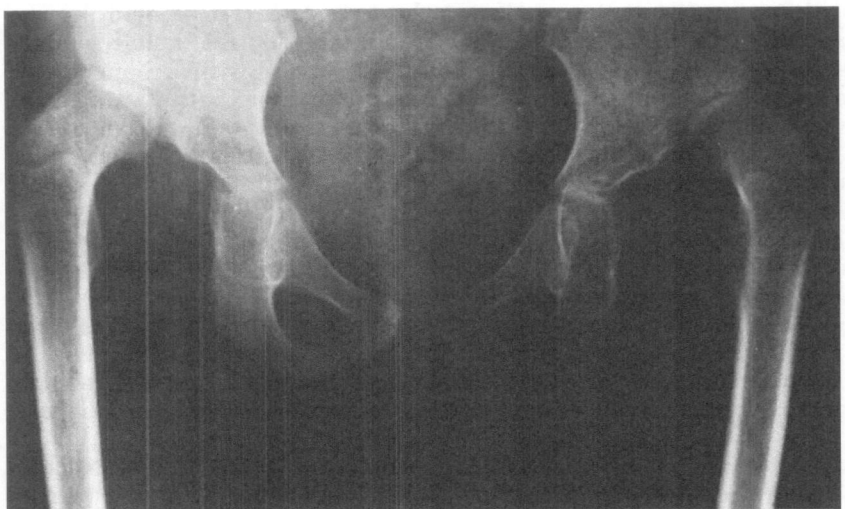

Fig. 3.13. Posterior dislocations in a child aged 4 years. The femoral heads are high and posterior and there is little chance of their grinding against the acetabular lip during flexion and extension

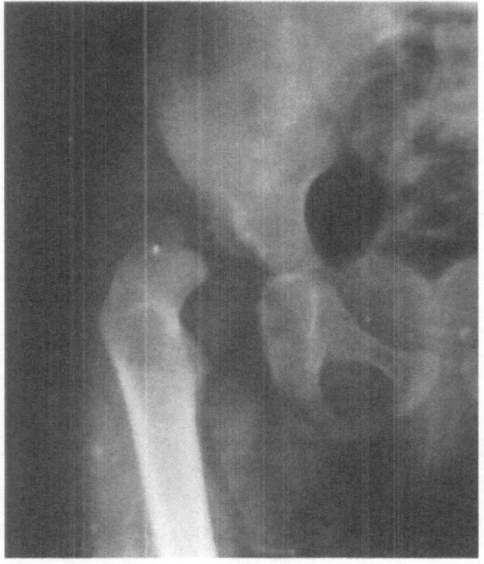

Fig. 3.14. With the head lodged on the lip of the acetabulum maximum damage will be done to the growing lip

UPPER END OF THE FEMUR

While there may be changes in the neck-shaft angle between one case and another, they are of only minor degree at birth and probably of no significance. The main deformity is to be found in the angle of anteversion. This may be as much as 45° or even 50° but may be as little as 0°; very occasionally there may be a few degrees of retroversion. As has already been suggested, it is those hips with the greater angle of anteversion which are more at risk.

The usual angle of anteversion at birth is about 25°–35°. In the presence of displacement the angle increases to 70°, 80°, or even 90° at times, so that there must be some mechanism which causes this increase. Figure 3.3 shows roughly the position of the upper end of the femur in relation to the pelvis in the usual dislocation. In this position the posterior aspect of the head and neck of the femur are against the hard wall of the pelvis, whereas the anterior aspect is only in contact with soft tissue. The leg lies in some lateral rotation and each time the child tries to rotate the leg medially pressure will be applied to the posterior aspect of the head and neck, which will mould it progressively into increasing anteversion because the upper end of the femur at this early age is growing rapidly and is very malleable.

In a subluxation the head of the femur never leaves the acetabulum, so the posterior aspect of the head is never in contact with the side of the pelvis. But with the hip in the subluxated position the leg lies in some lateral rotation, so that the posterior aspect of the head will be in contact with the anterior lip of the acetabulum and will be subject to pressure, which will be increased with every movement and further increased when the child begins to bear weight and stand, so that anteversion will increase just as quickly as if the hip were dislocated.

Anteversion seems to increase rapidly up to 70° and then more slowly up to 80°, and occasionally even up to 90°; by the time this degree of deformity is reached pressure on the posterior aspect of the head and neck will have become minimal. As will be mentioned later, under the influence of pressures induced by treatment the angle of anteversion may increase up to 160° or even 170° (p. 142).

REFERENCES

Haas J (1948) Congenital dislocation of the hip. Thomas, Springfield
Somerville EW (1953) Development of congenital dislocation of the hip. J Bone Joint Surg [Br] 35:568
Somerville EW (1974) The nature of the congenitally dislocated hip. Proc R Soc Med 67:1169
Trueta J (1957) The normal vascular anatomy of the human femoral head during growth. J Bone Joint Surg [Br] 39:358

4 Nine Months to Three-and-a-Half Years

DIAGNOSIS

In the age group 9 months to $3\frac{1}{2}$ years the clunk tests of Ortolani and Barlow are only rarely possible. The diagnosis is most commonly made at the age of about 20 months, by which time the child will have been walking long enough for an abnormality of gait to have been noticed. If the displacement is bilateral the diagnosis will be made about 4 months later, presumably because a bilateral limp will be less easily recognised than one which is unilateral.

Before the child has started walking it may have been noticed that the legs are asymmetrical. The affected leg will lie in some lateral rotation and may appear to be short. There may be a difference in the thigh and groin creases, in that they will be more pronounced on the dislocated side. These crease signs are unreliable because they may be present in normal babies, but when a dislocation is present the creases are commonly abnormal. As the child gets older the appearance of dislocation becomes less clear but the limp becomes more obvious.

Examination of the hip in extension shows that there is a firm round swelling just below and lateral to the anterior superior iliac spine. The child does not mind pressure on the spine but dislikes pressure on the swelling. When the hip is flexed the swelling disappears posteriorly into the buttock. The swelling is the head of the femur. Flexion and extension of the hip are full but abduction is usually restricted in both flexion and extension. Medial rotation is restricted but lateral rotation is increased. In this type of dislocation, which is by far the most common, there is no excessive lordosis in the lumbar spine.

The Trendelenberg test can only be used when the child is old enough to stand and to co-operate. It is therefore only of value in the older child, in whom it will usually be positive in the presence of a dislocation. But it is very easy to obtain a false-positive result because of nonco-operation.

In the very severe type of dislocation in which the displacement is posterosuperior the head of the femur will be palpable high in the buttock; the instability will be much greater; and a lordosis will develop, which may become severe. In this series this type of dislocation has not been seen in children under the age of 4 years and it has always been bilateral.

TREATMENT

To grow normally a joint must be mechanically sound. Once the structural changes which have been described have become established in either subluxation or dislocation they must be corrected if the joint is to be made mechanically sound. Treatment is in two phases: reduction and stabilisation (Somerville and Scott 1957).

Reduction

Because of the risk of damaging the blood supply to the ossific nucleus or of injuring the growth plate, all manoeuvres must be carried out with the greatest care and force must be avoided at all times. Any form of manipulative reduction involves a quite unacceptable risk and should not be attempted at any stage. The initial stage of reduction must be carried out with great gentleness and very slowly. There are several forms of traction which can be employed, usually with abduction. Having tried these other forms of reduction we have always come back to the use of the Wingfield frame as described by Scott (1953). This is a modification of the Jones abduction hip frame, which allows abduction of each hip to 90° (Fig 4.1). The basis is a strong iron frame onto which is fastened a soft leather-covered mattress filled with kapok and the legs of which are separated from the body to allow for very wide abduction. If frame reduction is to be used it is important to have nurses who are experienced in this method. Unless such people are available it is better to use another method.

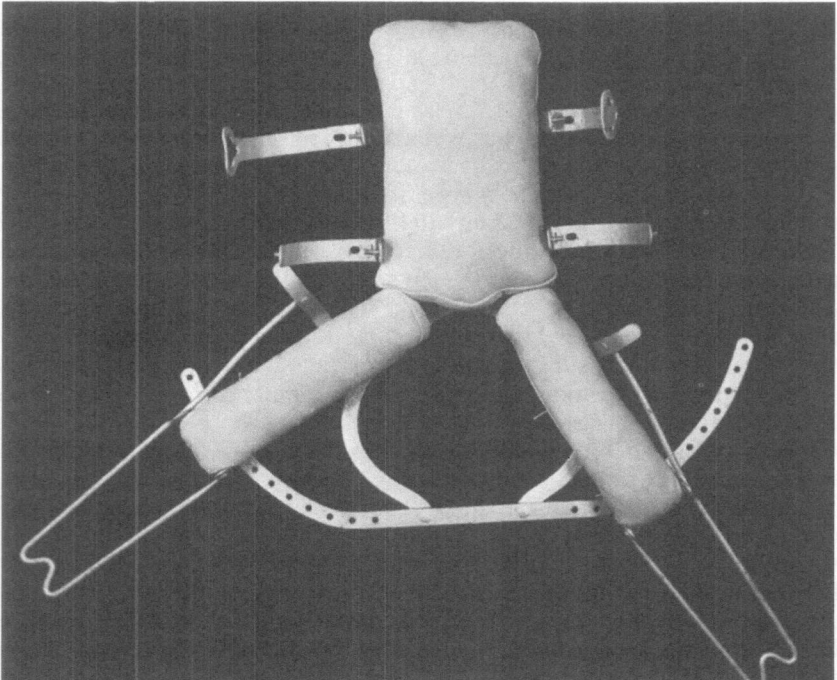

Fig. 4.1. The Wingfield frame. A modified Jones abduction frame which allows abduction of the hips to 90° on each side

The child is placed on the frame under sedation. Strapping extensions are applied to the legs to above the knees and the extension tapes are tied to the extension bows in such a way as to promote some medial rotation by passing the outer tape over the outside bar and the medial tape under the inner bar. At the knee, support must be placed behind the upper end of the tibia and never behind the lower end of the femur.

The legs are gently bandaged to the knock-knee bars, the bandage passing from without medially, and the legs are abducted 45° on each side. The frame is raised on wooden blocks to make nursing easier, and countertraction is applied by raising the foot of the bed. The legs are alternately abducted one hole each day until the angle between them is about 180° (Fig. 4.2). If during the course of this abduction the adductors become tight, which is not uncommon, the rate of abduction is slowed or stopped for a few days and is resumed when they have relaxed. In this age group it has very rarely been necessary to do an adductor tenotomy.

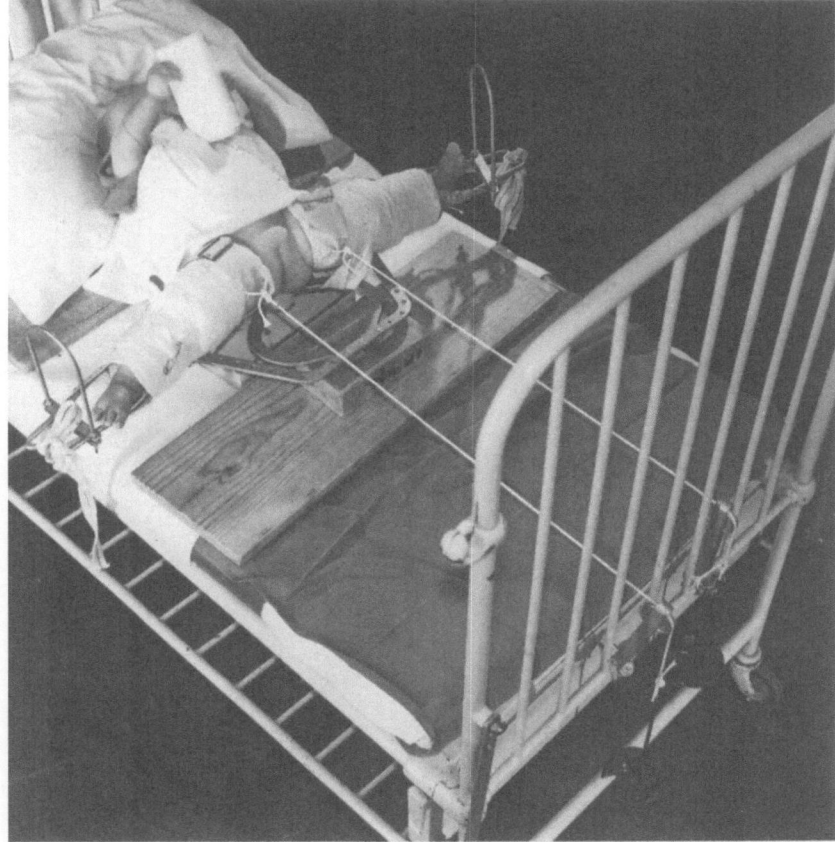

Fig. 4.2. Both hips are widely abducted with a cross-pull at right angles to each femur

In some cases the reduction of the femoral head down to the acetabulum is not achieved without a cross-pull. This is obtained by a sling, very well padded with sponge rubber, and applied as high as possible on the thigh. The pull must be at 90° to the thigh so that no strain will fall on the knee (Fig. 4.2). The pull, which is through a cord over a pulley, should not exceed 1½ lb.

Reduction of the head of the femur to the level of the acetabulum in a unilateral dislocation will take 3–4 weeks; in a bilateral dislocation 4–8 weeks is required, and in a subluxation, 7–10 days. The process must never be hurried to save time.

ARTHROGRAPHY

It is now necessary to determine whether the displacement is a subluxation (i.e., the limbus is not inverted and is not causing an obstruction) or a dislocation (i.e., the limbus is inverted and is causing an obstruction to concentric reduction). This can be done with certainty only by means of arthrography (Mitchel 1963).

In the early cases arthrography was performed before the child was placed on the frame and again when reduction of the femoral head to the acetabulum had been achieved. Arthrography before traction was later discontinued because it so consistently showed the limbus to be inverted in all dislocations (Fig. 4.3), and it is of more importance to know whether or not the limbus is causing an obstruction after the head has been pulled down.

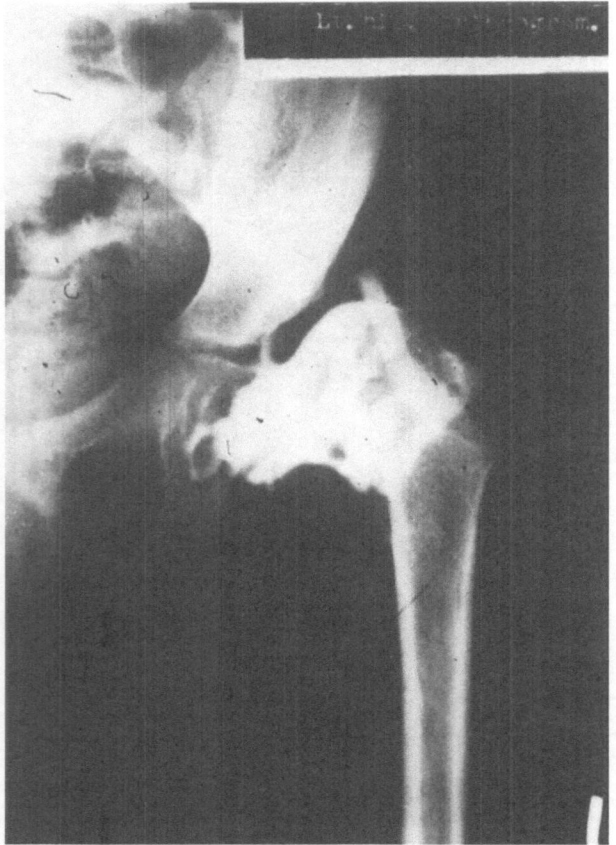

Fig. 4.3. An arthrogram of a dislocated hip before treatment was started, showing that the limbus is already inverted

Technique

Under anaesthesia, the child is removed from the frame in the operating theatre and the hip is prepared in the usual way. The femoral pulse is palpated in front of the hip joint. A fine needle with a short bevel is introduced just lateral to the femoral artery and just below the inguinal ligament down to the head of the femur. The needle will pass through the capsule and into the cartilage of the femoral head, so that when the head is gently rotated the tip of the needle will move one way with the head and the butt end will move the other way—that is, in the opposite direction to the rotation of the leg. If the butt moves the same way as the leg the point of the needle is not in the head. While pressure is applied to the plunger of the syringe the needle is gently withdrawn. When the bevel of the needle enters the joint space the dye will run in easily. If there is difficulty in finding the space between the capsule and the head, which is only a potential space, traction on the leg will cause relaxation of the capsule and make the procedure simpler. A 15% solution of radio-opaque dye is injected. The only true test that the injection is being made into the joint is that the fluid, having been injected, can be sucked back again. This is done several times, to ensure that the whole joint is filled. A volume of 3–4 ml is left in the joint, according to the size of the child. The fluid left in should never be under tension. It has been suggested that arthrography may lead to vascular damage, but in this series no single instance of this has been seen.

An alternative method of injection is through the adductor region. In some ways this is simpler, but has not been practised in this series because of the possible risk of infection. The use of an image intensifier makes the procedure easier.

The only radiographic view which is of value is the anteroposterior; lateral radiographs are of no value.

Interpretation

In the normal hip the femoral head can be seen outlined by a thin layer of opaque fluid (Fig. 4.4). It fits accurately into the acetabulum. The lip of the acetabulum is

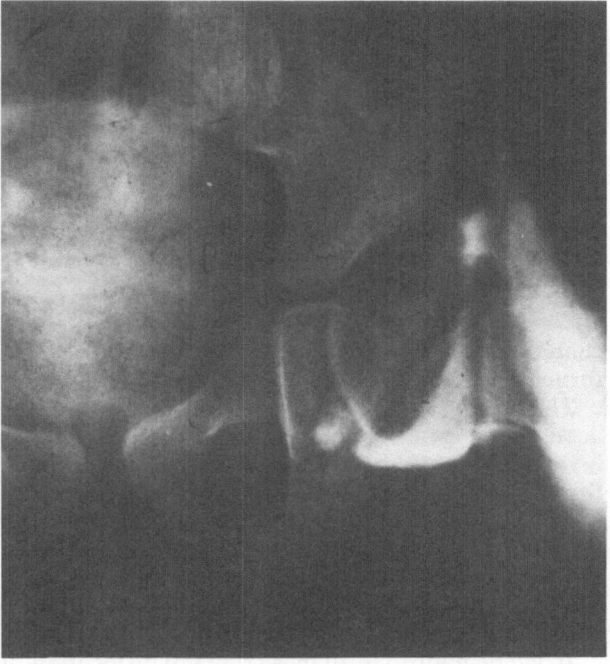

Fig. 4.4. Arthrogram of a normal hip. The joint is outlined by a very thin line of opaque medium

defined as a sharp point with the capsule attached about ⅛ in. from the tip, forming the typical appearance of the limbic thorn.

In the case of a subluxation, when the leg is lying free, i.e., in some lateral rotation, the head of the femur will fit loosely and the dye will appear like a moon at the end of the first quarter (Fig. 4.5), but there is no obstruction. If the subluxation is of long

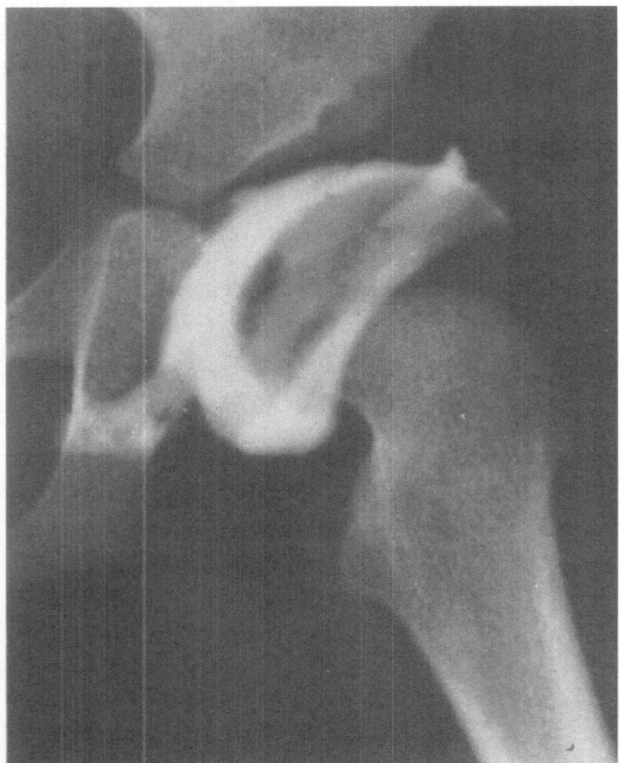

Fig. 4.5. Arthrogram of a subluxated hip showing the crescent of dye. The limbus is slightly everted but there is no suggestion of inversion or obstruction

standing it can be seen that there is distortion of the lip of the acetabulum, which is turned out, rendering the acetabulum defective (Fig. 4.6).

The appearance of a dislocation is quite different. The lip or limbus of the acetabulum is turned into the joint. While the posterior part of the limbus is always inverted, very often the superior part is also inverted, and in an arthrogram it is only this superior part which is seen (Fig. 4.7). Sometimes the deformity is all posterior, when the limbus cannot be seen, but it is obvious that there is an obstruction because the head does not fit into the acetabulum centrally. If the inverted limbus is very large the appearance may be misleading because it will fill the whole floor of the acetabulum and it may be difficult to see the outline of it (Fig. 4.8), but it will be clear that the head is not fitting correctly.

It will be noticed in all these types of dislocation that when the head of the femur is reduced to the level of the acetabulum there is pooling of the dye in the floor,

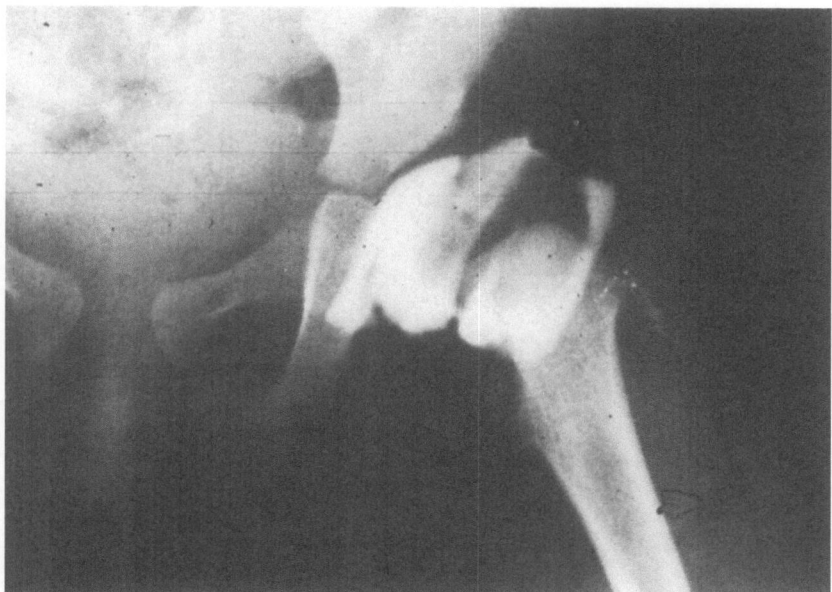

Fig. 4.6. Arthrogram of a severe subluxation showing deformity of the limbus, which is being flattened out of the joint

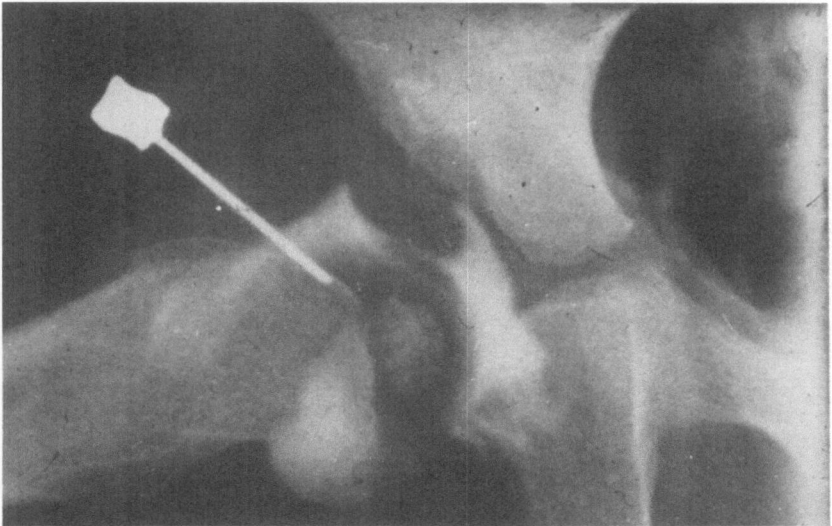

Fig. 4.7. Arthrogram of a dislocated hip in wide abduction. It can be clearly seen how the inverted limbus is preventing concentric reduction

indicating that the obstruction cannot be deep in the acetabulum but must be at the periphery (Fig. 4.9).

The appearance of the inverted limbus may vary greatly, as is shown diagrammatically in Figs. 4.10 and 4.11. Figure 4.10 shows the state before the head has been reduced to the acetabulum, and Fig. 4.11 afterwards.

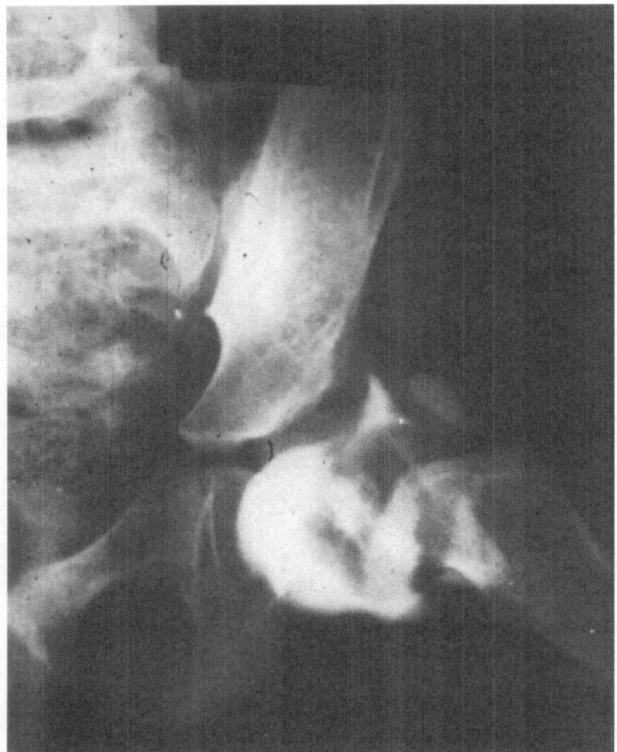

Fig. 4.8. Arthrogram of a very large limbus, which is flattened into the floor of the acetabulum

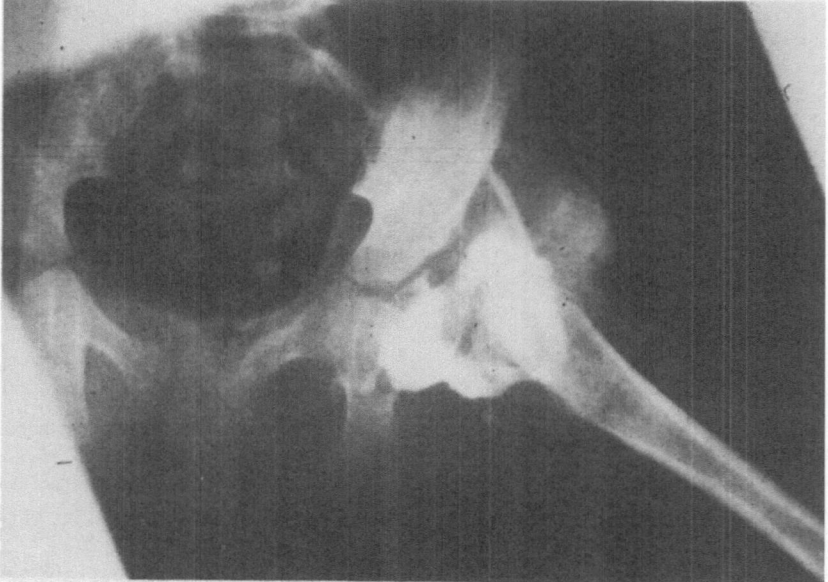

Fig. 4.9. Arthrogram of a dislocated hip, showing the limbus compressed against the roof of the acetabulum when the hip is abducted

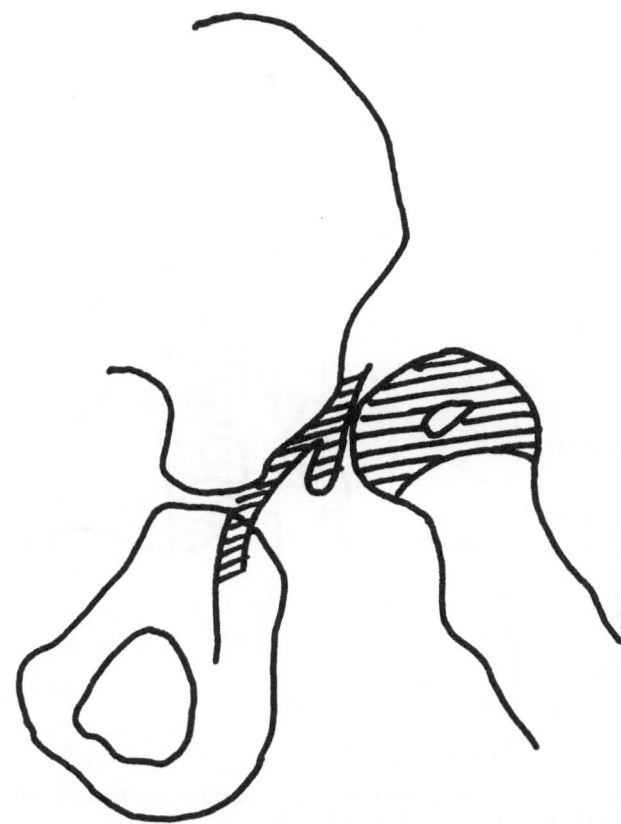

Fig. 4.10 Tracing of an arthrogram of a hip before the head has been reduced to the level of the acetabulum

It has been suggested (Severin 1941, 1950) that if the head is maintained opposite the acetabulum for long enough it will force its way in. This is sometimes the case, but it will all too often be at the expense of a false reduction (Fig. 4.12), with inevitable damage to the growing lip of the acetabulum leading almost certainly to deterioration later.

SUBLUXATION

For the purpose of obtaining reduction, subluxation and dislocation are treated differently. In cases of subluxation there is no obstruction but it is still necessary to obtain full medial rotation of the leg to neutralise the excessive anteversion. Under the anaesthetic used for the arthrography a plastic spica is applied with the femur abducted 45° and in as much internal rotation as is possible without using force—usually about 45°. Two weeks later the same procedure is repeated, when full, i.e. about 90°, medial rotation will be possible without difficulty and the spica will be reapplied in this position. This is retained for 2 weeks.

It should be noted that with the hip in medial rotation 45° of abduction of the femur is not the same as 45° of abduction of the leg (Fig. 4.13), and due allowance must be made for this. In unilateral displacement the other hip is always included in the plaster, which is extended to the knee, to make nursing easier and to prevent

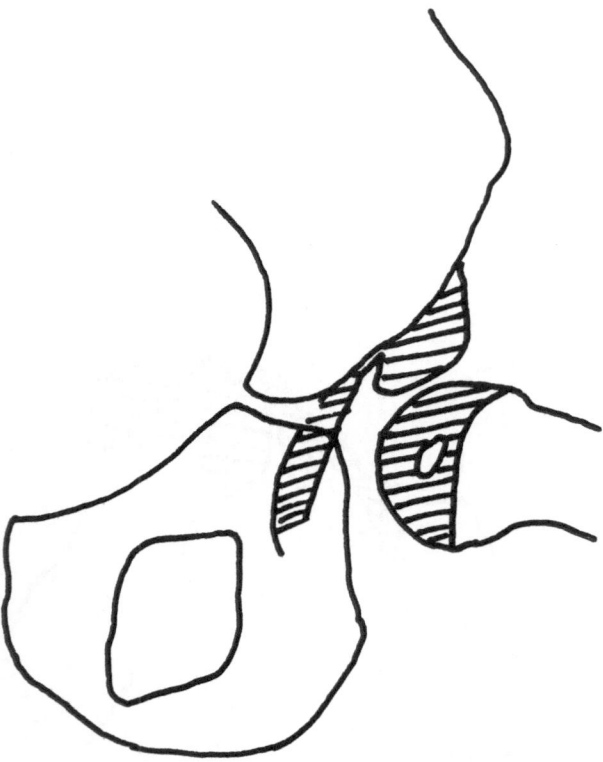

Fig. 4.11. Tracing of an arthrogram of the same hip after the hip has been 'reduced'. The inverted limbus can be seen preventing true reduction

adduction; this is because adduction of the young hip will affect the development of the joint, leading to subluxation or in extreme cases dislocation if allowed to continue long enough. (Fig. 4.14).

DISLOCATION

Correct concentric reduction of a dislocated hip will involve removal of the obstructing limbus by one means or another. In this series it has been the custom to excise it whenever arthrography has demonstrated that it is causing an obstruction.

Excision of the Limbus

The operation is carried out through a slightly oblique transverse incision (Somerville 1953) 2½ in. in length centred ¾ in. below the anterior superior iliac spine (Fig. 4.15), with the child lying supine. The space between the sartorius and tensor fascia lata is opened up and the anterior 1 in. of the tensor muscle is divided close to the iliac crest. It is better not to strip it off subperiosteally. The anterior margin of the ilium is then followed down to the rectus muscle with its reflected head and the white shining capsule, which is cleared of fat so that all the structures are well defined. The rectus is separated from the capsule, to which it is sometimes adherent, and if the reflected head is large it is divided transversely. A bone lever is passed between the

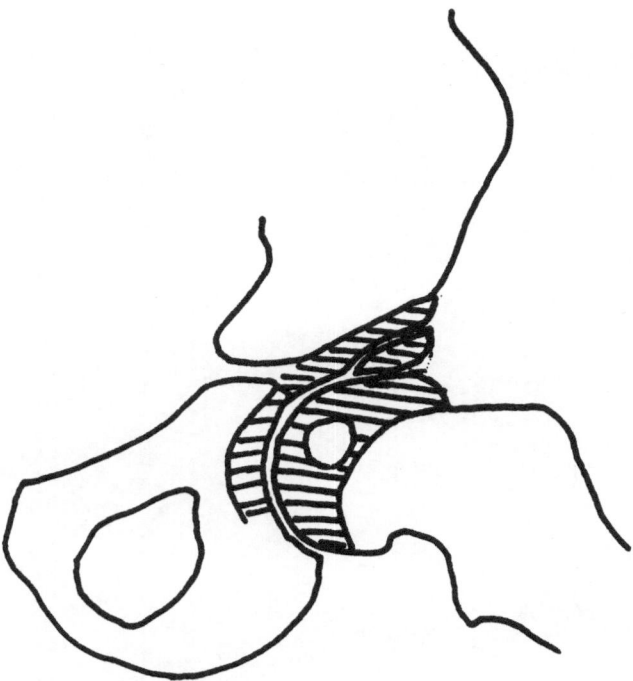

Fig. 4.12. If the head of the femur is allowed to press on the inverted limbus for long enough it will gradually reach the floor of the acetabulum. But the reduction will be a false one and may cause lasting damage to the growth potential of the joint

capsule and the rectus across the front of the joint and down the medial side. A transverse incision is made in the capsule as close as is reasonably possible to the lip of the acetabulum, care being taken not to damage the lip. This incision is carried from the posterosuperior part of the joint across the front and down the medial side as far as is possible, at the same time dividing the transverse ligament, which in the older child may be tight. This incision is rendered quick and safe by the bone lever; the incision on the medial side is made onto the lever, which keeps the important structures out of the way.

The bone lever is removed and is replaced by a small Langenbeck's retractor, with which the rectus is lifted forwards. Traction is applied to the leg by an assistant to pull the head of the femur out of the acetabulum by about ½ in., permitting easy examination of the inside of the joint. Usually the inverted limbus will be seen quite easily, looking rather like a medial meniscus. A blunt hook is passed round it, the tip being brought out through the base. Keeping tension on the hook the limbus, anterior to the hook, is detached with a scalpel until the hook comes out. The free end is grasped with a small Kocher's forceps and with tension on it the posterior part is detached with curved scissors, the inner blade of which is passed down inside the capsule (Fig. 4.16). After an inspection of the inside of the joint traction on the leg is stopped and the leg is rotated medially through 90°, which will reduce the head into the acetabulum and close the gap in the capsule so that no suture is needed except to reattach the tensor fascia lata to the iliac crest.

The two important things in this operation are to clear the capsule and define the rectus and its reflected head before proceeding, and to make the transverse incision

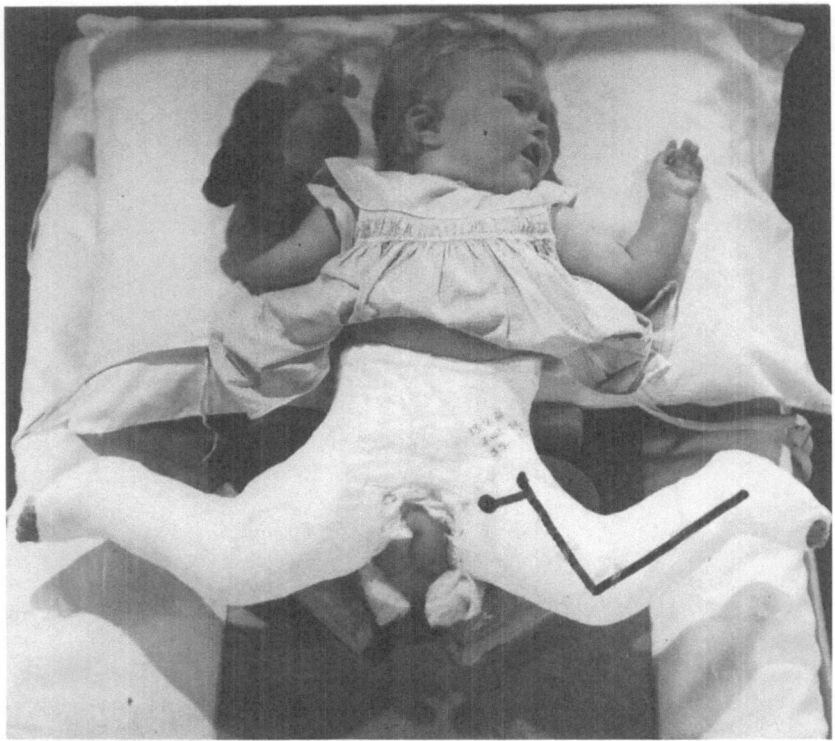

Fig. 4.13. This photograph shows why apparent abduction may be considerably greater than the real abduction when the hip is in full internal rotation

in the capsule close to the acetabular lip. Failure to do so can make a relatively simple operation difficult.

After closure of the wound a 1½ spica is applied (Fig. 4.14), i.e., including the whole of one leg and the other one to the knee. If both hips are dislocated the operation can be performed on both sides at the same time. It is not an operation which causes shock and a young age is not a contraindication

The plaster spica is retained for 1 month, during which time, if the mother has learned how to nurse the child in plaster, the patient can be taken home on a wooden frame, which makes nursing easier. The child should always be kept with the head slightly raised, to prevent urine from getting down inside the plaster.

Stabilisation

Whether the initial condition was a subluxation or a dislocation the stabilisation procedure is the same: normal mechanics is restored to the hip by means of a high femoral osteotomy.

In the earlier cases in this series the osteotomy was purely rotational, to correct anteversion. The problem has always been to estimate the angle of anteversion. Radiological techniques provide some degree of accuracy when the development of the upper end of the femur is nearing completion. But in the very young child, with

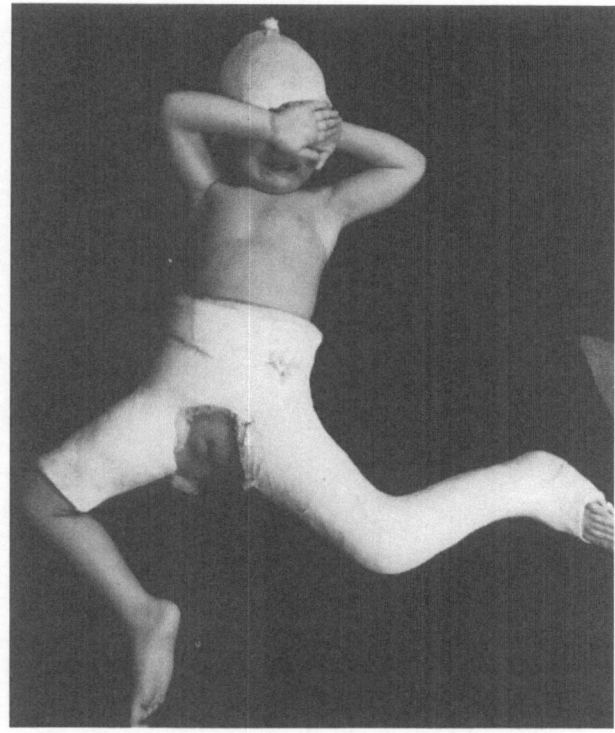

Fig. 4.14. This photograph shows the position in a 1½ plaster spica after reduction for unilateral displacement

the upper end of the femur still partly cartilaginous, the measurements are likely to be inaccurate. One essential point of measurement is the centre of the head of the femur, which is taken to be the centre of the ossific nucleus which is all that is visible, the assumption being that the nucleus is in the centre of the head. This is not a warrantable assumption as it usually is not central (p. 30).

Trial and error have shown that over all, the best results are obtained with a rotational correction of 70°. It also seems that an addition of 10°–15° of varus at the osteotomy improves stability still further and improves early mobilisation and walking for reasons which are explained later (p. 97) (Somerville 1978).

TECHNIQUE

High femoral osteotomy is performed with the child in the supine position. The leg is held in full medial rotation while an incision about 4 in. long is made from the prominence of the trochanter downwards. The direction of the incision is slightly forwards, so that after the leg has been rotated it will become vertical. The fascia is split longitudinally. The muscle fibres are separated by blunt dissection down to the bone. This reduces bleeding and therefore ischaemia, fibrosis, and stiffness. The periosteum is incised in length and the bone exposed with bone levers anteriorly and posteriorly so that the periosteum is preserved as a tube.

The lower edge of the cartilaginous trochanter is defined and a $^7/_{64}$ in. Steinmann pin

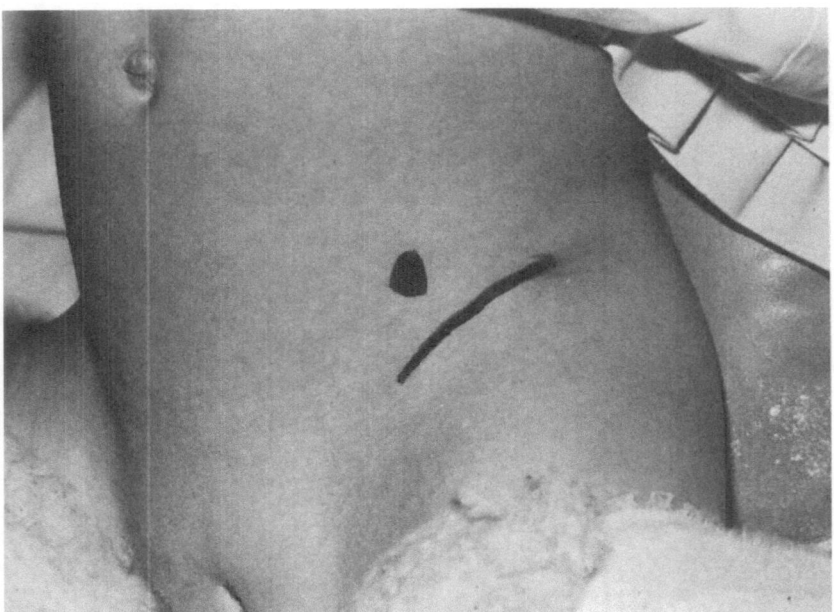

Fig. 4.15. The incision used for excision of the limbus. A transverse or slightly oblique incision will heal very much better than a vertical incision. A Smith–Petersen type of incision should not be used in children

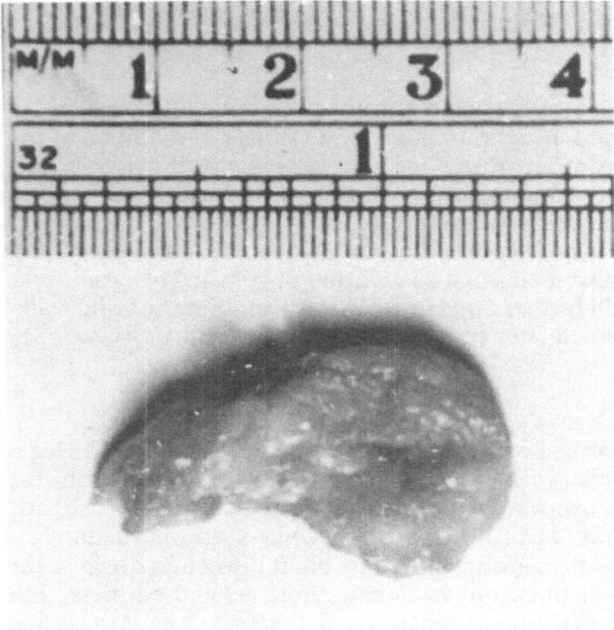

Fig. 4.16. A typical limbus which has been excised

is introduced just below it. The pin is covered by a guard to prevent too-deep penetration (Fig. 4.17). Care must be taken to ensure that the pin is introduced into the lateral aspect of the bone and passes through the diameter (Fig. 4.18). A small

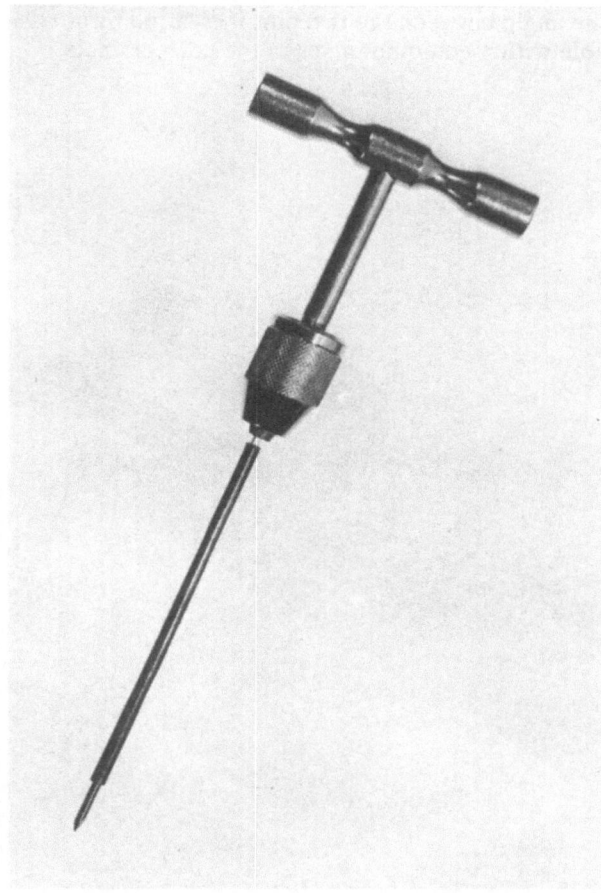

Fig. 4.17. The 7/64 in. Steinmann's pin with introducer and guard.

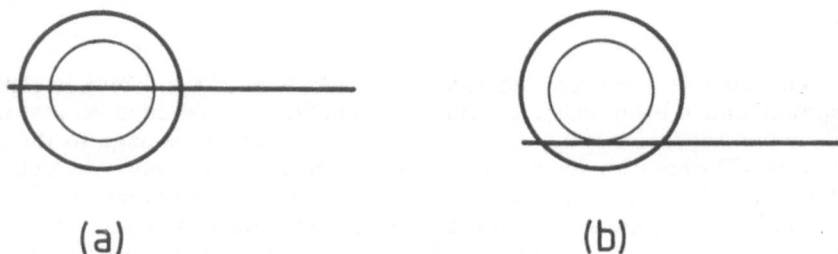

(a)   **(b)**

Fig. 4.18. This diagram emphasises the importance of the pin passing through the diameter of the bone. Failure to achieve this will cause a considerable increase or decrease in the rotation obtained

plate is threaded onto the pin through its upper hole and is laid along the bone (Fig. 4.19). A second pin is introduced opposite the upper hole in the lower half of the plate and anterior to it so that the rotation will be lateral. It is introduced at an angle of 70° to the upper pin, again great care being taken to ensure that it passes through the diameter of the bone, as otherwise the plate will not fit correctly after rotation. The angle between the two pins is ensured by an assistant standing at the foot of the table with a goniometer set to the correct angle.

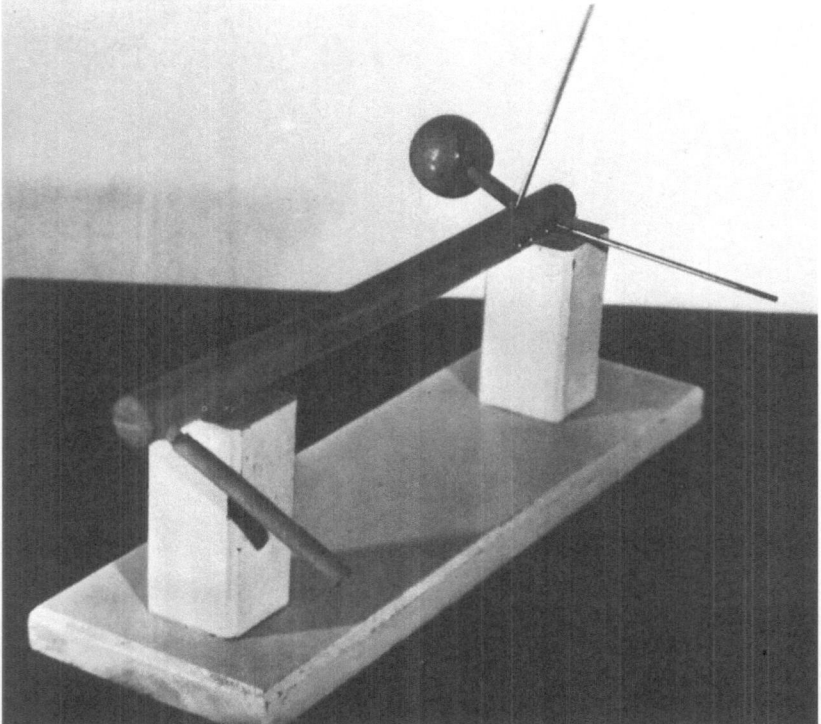

Fig. 4.19. In the model the upper pin has been introduced into the lateral apsect of the upper end of the femur. The plate has been slotted onto it through its upper hole. The lower pin has been introduced opposite the upper hole in the lower half of the plate and at an angle of 70° to the upper one

The plate is removed and the bone lever behind the femur is replaced by a spatula-ended lever which is turned through 90°, i.e., on edge, so that muscles are detached subperiosteally at the linea aspera, avoiding damage to the perforating arteries. The anterior lever is also turned on edge and the bone is divided with a hand saw ½ in. proximal to the lower pin, keeping the periosteum intact.

The lower fragment is rotated laterally until the pins are parallel when the plate is threaded onto them. The lowest hole is then drilled and the screw is introduced. It is important to drill the lower hole first because it ensures that the plate will be in the correct position. The empty hole in the upper part is similarly treated. The lower pin

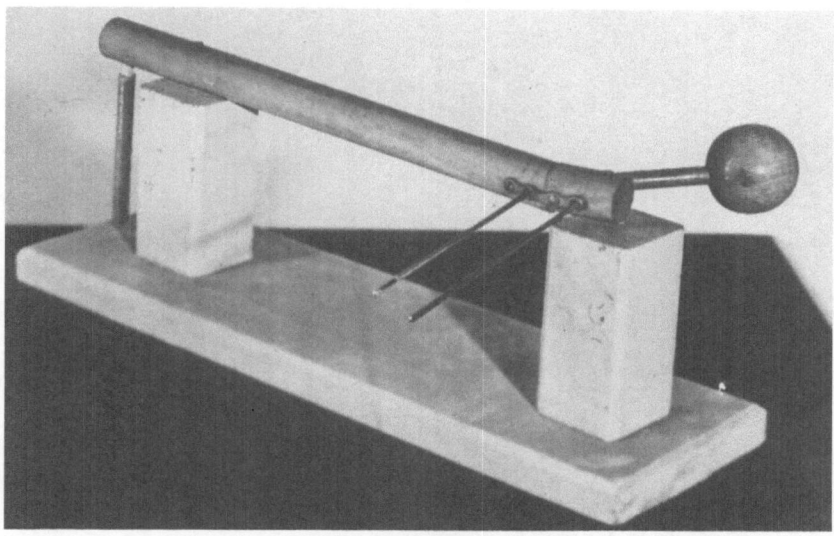

Fig. 4.20. The bone has been divided just above the lower pin and the lower fragment rotated until the pins are parallel and the plate is screwed in position. The two pins will now be removed one at a time and the screwing completed

is removed and a screw introduced into its track, which should be of the correct size so that further drilling will be unnecessary (Fig. 4.20). Lastly the upper pin is removed and the screw inserted. The muscle edges are lightly opposed and the fascia lata lightly closed as a separate layer before closure of the skin.

It is now routine to include 10°–15° of varus with the rotation at the site of the osteotomy. This requires a slight alteration in technique, which in some ways makes the operation simpler because the fragments when reduced are more stable.

The lower pin is used as a handle and the lower fragment is drawn out of the wound (Fig. 4.21); and with gouge-ended nibblers the cortex is nibbled away on the medial side of the bone where the point of the pin is protruding. Sufficient bone is removed to produce an angle of about 15° when the bone is rotated and the pins are in the same plane. Because of the natural flare of the greater trochanter, with this degree of angulation the outer border of the femur will often be straight, so that a straight plate can be applied and still obtain the required angulation (Figs. 4.22 and 4.23). Cosmetically this is much better than an obvious angulation. If the flare is insufficient the plate must be angled accordingly. The plate is threaded onto the two pins and fixed as described for simple rotation osteotomy. In either type of osteotomy the top screw should be $\frac{1}{4}$ in. longer than the others, because it will have gone into the base of the neck. After closure of the wound in layers a $1\frac{1}{2}$ spica is applied and retained for 6 weeks. After 6 weeks the osteotomy will be united and the child will be allowed to move about freely and walk as soon as possible, regardless of the radiological appearance.

It will be found that following a simple rotation osteotomy of 70° the leg will lie in some lateral rotation, and this position will continue for a while after walking has started. These slight difficulties can be overcome by the addition of the small amount

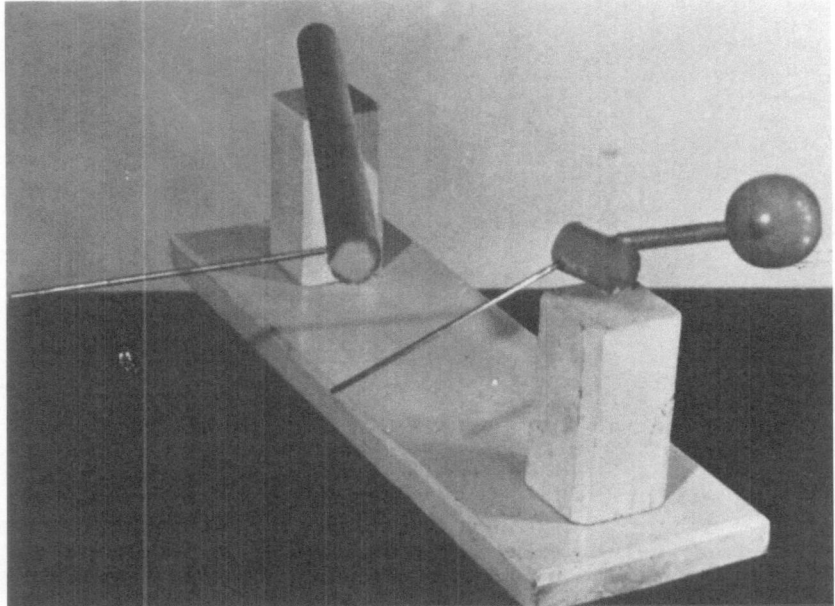

Fig. 4.21. If the osteotomy is to be made varus the lower fragment is drawn out of the wound and the medial cortex, which is where the tip of the lower pin will emerge, is removed with nibblers

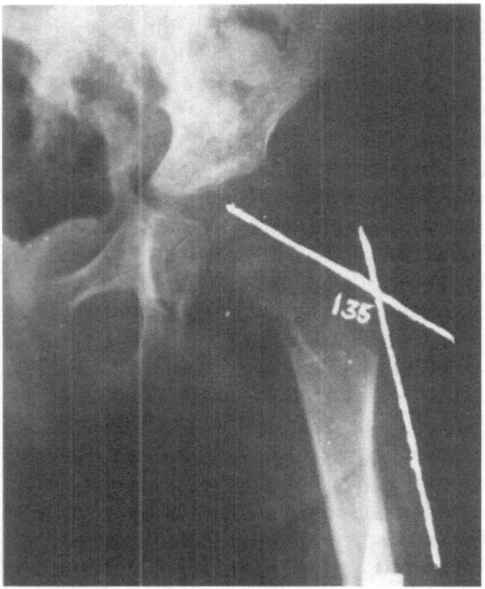

Fig. 4.22. The amount of flare of the greater trochanter can be seen

of varus; following the operation the leg will lie in a neutral rotation, and when walking is started the foot will be held to the front. The reason for this will be explained later (p. 97).

Figures 4.24–4.32 show a series of radiographs depicting the stages of treatment. It is desirable that the different stages of treatment should be carried out as a routine. The period of frame reduction must never be hurried, but once reduction has been achieved the subsequent stages should be carried out on schedule. The arthrography is carried out a few days later, followed immediately by excision of the limbus when indicated. The plaster is retained for 1 month; then the osteotomy is carried out and followed by a further 6 weeks in plaster before mobilisation is commenced. It has always proved safe to do the osteotomy 1 month after excision of the limbus and it may be safe to do it earlier, just as the osteotomy may be united well before 6 weeks and probably is, but it is better not to take the plaster off just to find out. Keeping to a routine means the parents know exactly what to expect and can make the necessary arrangements to take the child home after each operation.

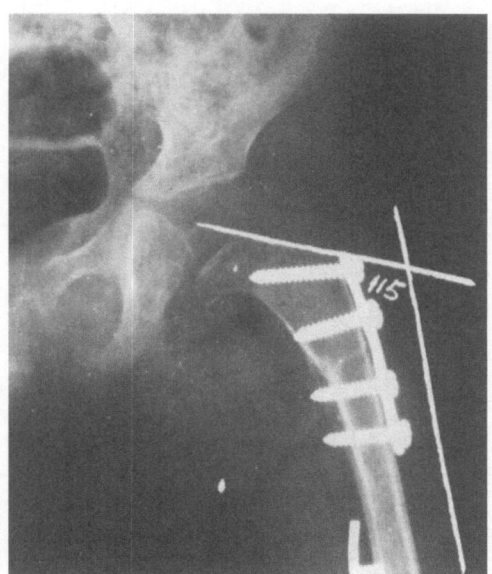

Fig. 4.23. The flare of the greater trochanter can be used to produce 20° of varus with minimal apparent angulation

BILATERAL DISLOCATIONS

In the treatment of bilateral dislocations the principles are the same as in the unilateral cases, but there are some differences in detail. Reduction on the frame will take longer at 4–8 weeks. If reduction has not been achieved by then a formal open reduction should be carried out with, if necessary, shortening of the femoral shaft.

Excision of the limbus or open reductions are not operations that cause shock in the patients, and they can be carried out on the two sides at the same time, but osteotomies do cause some shock and should not be carried out on both sides at the same time unless the child is aged more than 2 years. Otherwise there should be an interval of a week between the two operations.

The most important consideration is during the period of mobilisation. It is very important that both hips should mobilise at the same speed. If one mobilises rapidly but there is a persistence of abduction on the other, then the one that mobilises quickly will adduct and subluxate, or in extreme cases even dislocate. If persistence of abduction is of a minor degree only, even as little as 5°–10°, the development of the other hip may be seriously impaired.

These children should be kept in hospital under observation until it is clear that adduction is taking place equally on the two sides, even though it may be slow. If it is not, then the hip which is mobilising rapidly must be immobilised in a hip spica until the other one has caught up.

Mobilisation of bilaterally dislocated hips is always much slower than mobilisation of unilateral displacement, and it takes longer for the child to learn to walk.

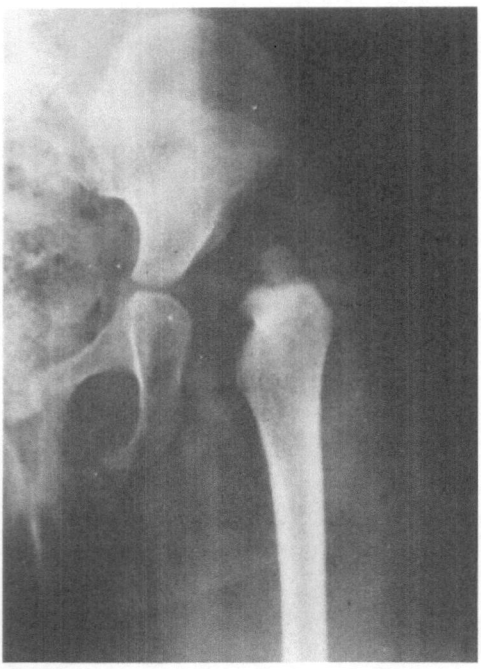

Fig. 4.24. Typical dislocation of the hip in a child aged 20 months

THE PARENTS

It is of the greatest importance that the parents should be taken fully into the surgeon's confidence before treatment. The steps of treatment must be clearly explained and the dates of each stage decided. It is desirable for the mother to spend as much time as possible in the ward looking after the child so that she will be competent to nurse the child at home between admissions. It is important to stress the point that treatment does not end with discharge from hospital. The hip has a long way to grow and has got off to a bad start. Follow-up is essential until the end of growth and as far beyond as possible to ensure that normal growth has been achieved and is continuing; and if it is not, then some surgical adjustment may have to be made to correct it. If the parents have been forewarned of this it will make the explanations much easier should it become necessary.

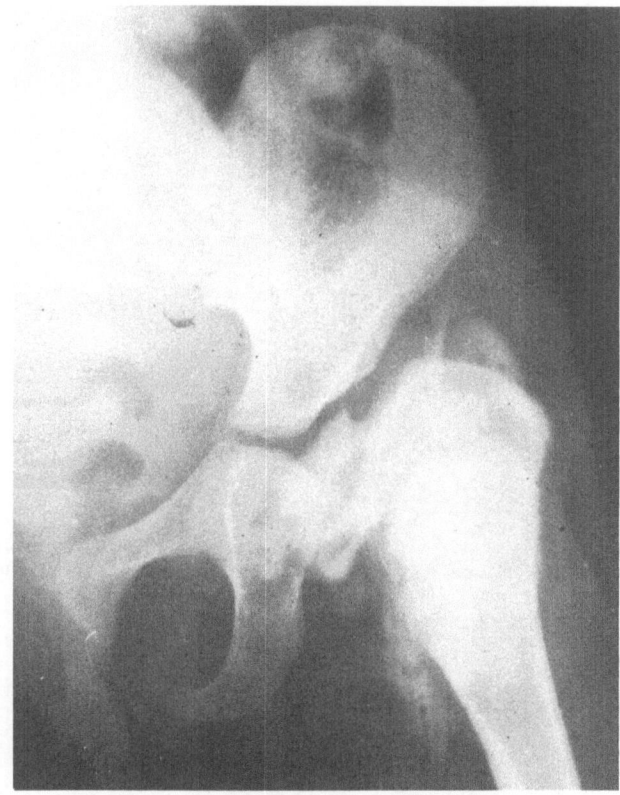

Fig. 4.25. The arthrogram before treatment of the hip illustrated in Fig 4.24 shows the inverted limbus

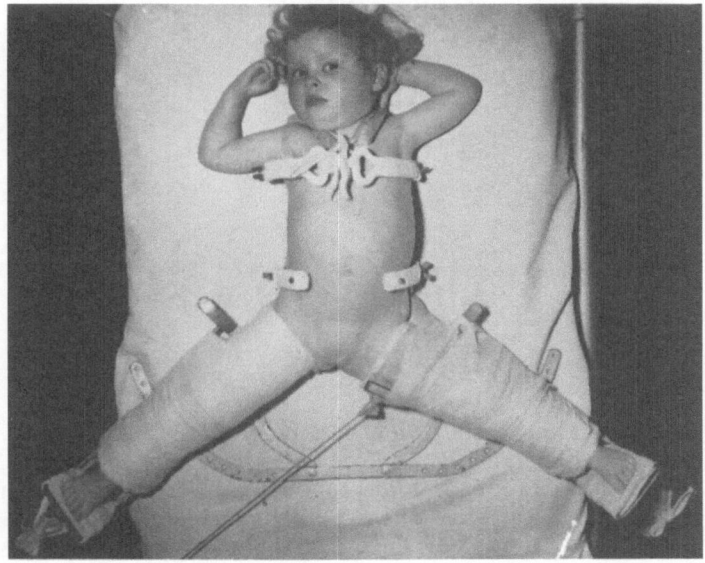

Fig. 4.26. The
position on the frame

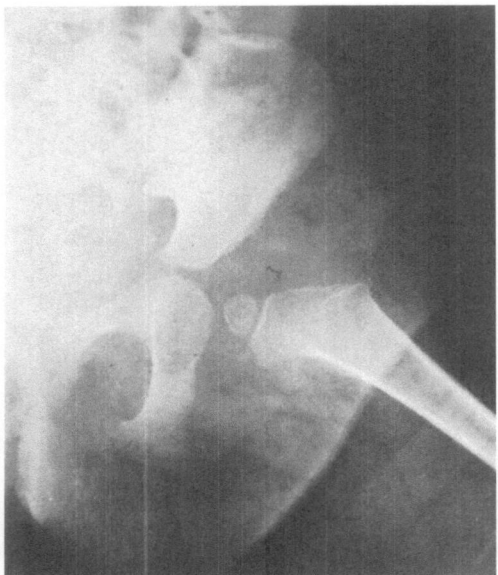

Fig. 4.27. The head is pulled down to the acetabulum but is still standing out. This position must not be mistaken for reduction

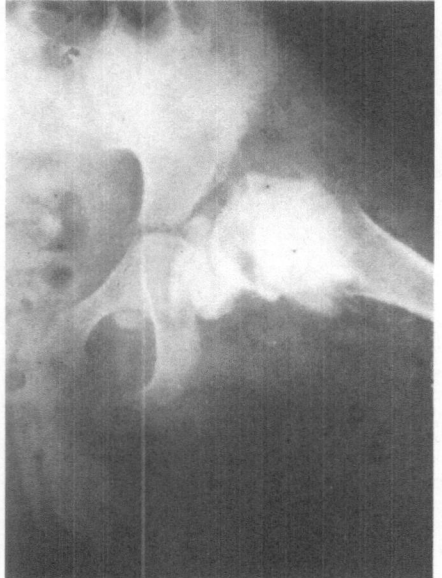

Fig. 4.28. An arthrogram of the same hip as in Fig. 4.27 shows the true position, with the inverted limbus and pooling

MEDIUM LONG-TERM REVIEW

A medium long-term review was undertaken early in 1974. In all, 177 hips in 144 patients, treated along the lines described, were examined. The hips were selected from a total of about 450. The follow-up was for a minimum period of 10 years and a maximum of 25. Most of the patients had been seen at yearly intervals since the conclusion of treatment. The age at the time of treatment was between 9 months and

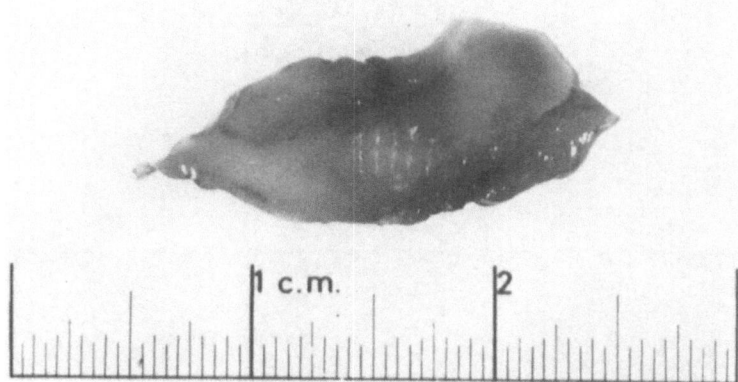

Fig. 4.29. The limbus which was excised

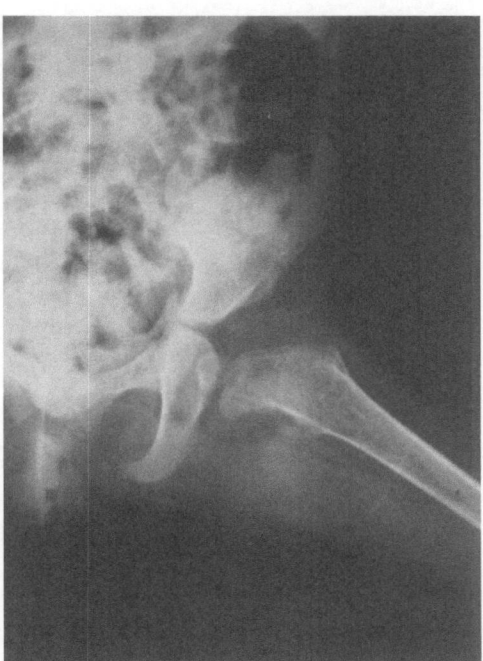

Fig. 4.30. After the limbus has been excised it is seen that the head is now well placed in the acetabulum. The fact that it appears a little lower is good. (Compare with Fig. 4.27.)

$3\frac{1}{2}$ years and none had previously been treated. The differentiation between dislocation and subluxation was made by arthrography.

Functional Assessment

The value of functional assessment in the early years after treatment is limited, because it is so often misleading. Many hips which are functionally good for many

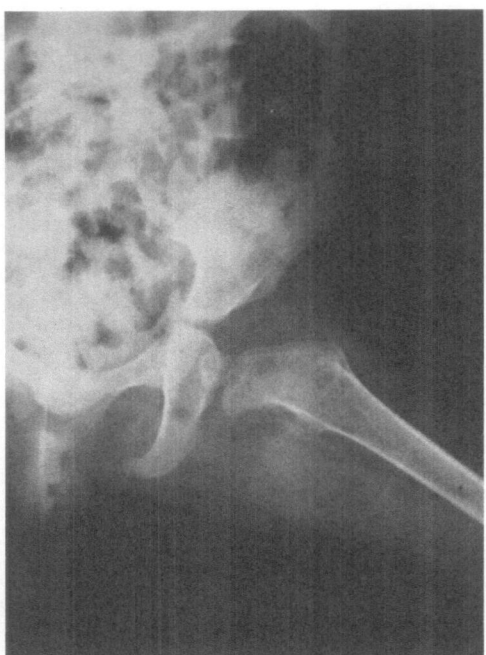

Fig. 4.31. The position is shown 6 weeks after rotation osteotomy of 70° at the time when the plaster was removed. Mobilisation was started 14 weeks after treatment began

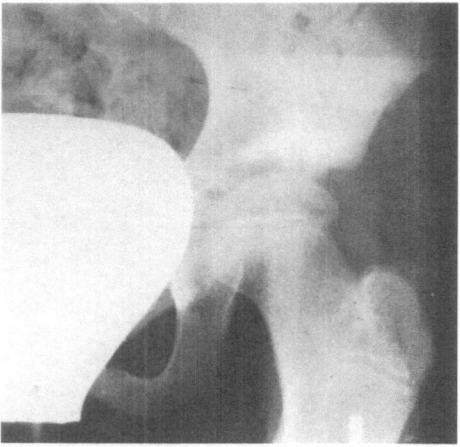

Fig. 4.32. Ten years later the condition of the hip shown in Fig. 4.31 is now acceptable

years are anatomically unacceptable, but in later years it becomes of greater significance. In the very long term it is the functional result which is all-important, regardless of the shape of the joint. It is more than likely that some hips with residual dysplasia will out-last those with an acetabulum which is too well developed.

Of the 144 patients, five had a severe limp, four had a moderate limp, and six a slight limp. Movement presented no problem; in no hip was flexion less than 90° and in only four was it less than 120°. Pain was unusual but ten had some pain with limited activity and in one it was sufficient to warrant a Chiari osteotomy. In some the plate caused a persistent ache which must not be confused with hip pain, and when the plate was removed the ache was relieved.

In 111 patients with unilateral displacement persistent foetal alignment was present in the other hip in 20. There were only two cases of true osteochondritis, which is interesting in view of other hips treated previously, in which the incidence was appreciably higher.

Radiological Assessment

To avoid going into too great detail the hips have been divided into three groups: Those that were considered to be acceptable; those that were unacceptable; and a small group in between, in which there was a minor degree of subluxation but which were giving no trouble and which after sometimes more than 20 years were showing no sign of deterioration. Such hips are obviously too good to be called failures but not good enough to be claimed as successes. Subsequent investigation suggests that some of these will last longer than some of those with a well-formed acetabulum.

ACCEPTABLE

To be acceptable a hip must have a well-developed acetabulum with a CE angle of 20° or more and a congruous femoral head, and in a series of radiographs there must be no evidence of deterioration. In the case of bilateral dislocations it was not necessary for the two hips to look the same provided they complied with these criteria.

UNACCEPTABLE

Unacceptable hips show evidence of frank subluxation with evidence in serial radiographs of progressive deterioration and development of degenerative changes. Even in these unsatisfactory hips it was surprising how many of them were clinically good.

Table 4.1. General statistics

Unilateral dislocations	101	Right 23; left 88
Unilateral subluxations	10	
Bilateral displacement	66	
	177 (144 patients)	

Table 4.1 shows the overall distribution of the hips examined, and Fig. 4.33 the age distribution in unilateral and bilateral displacements.

UNILATERAL DISPLACEMENT

There were 101 unilateral dislocations examined and the overall results, disregarding age, showed that 80% were acceptable and 10% were unacceptable.

Table 4.2. Unilateral dislocations: overall results

Acceptable	80%
Minor subluxation	10%
Unacceptable	10%

The influence of age was well marked. In the youngest group (9–15 months of age) all the hips were acceptable at the time of examination. In the intermediate age group of 15–36 months 80% were acceptable and 12% were unacceptable, but in the group aged from 36 months to 42 months there was a fall to 66% acceptable and 24% unacceptable.

There were only ten hips with unilateral subluxation, and all were treated below the age of 2 years. Nine had results which were acceptable.

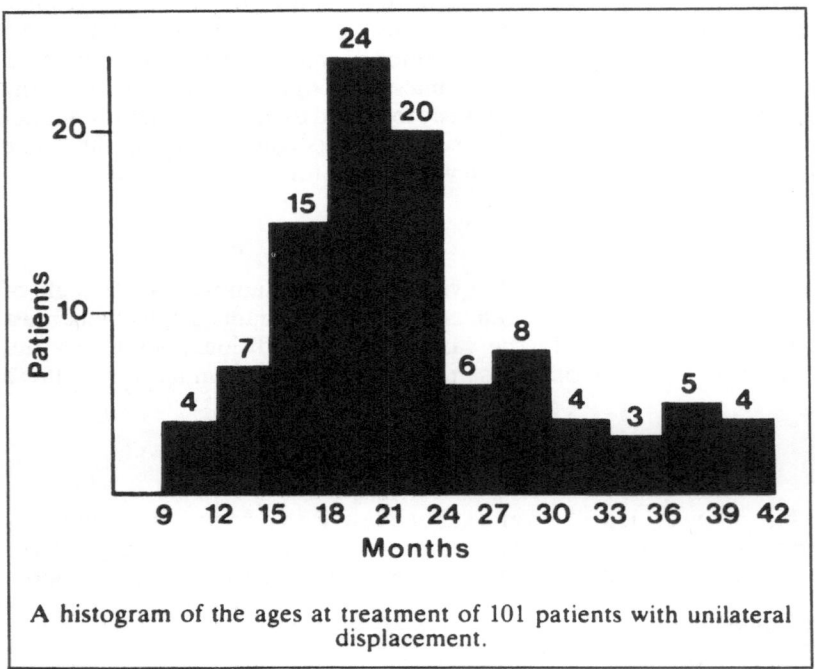

A histogram of the ages at treatment of 101 patients with unilateral displacement.

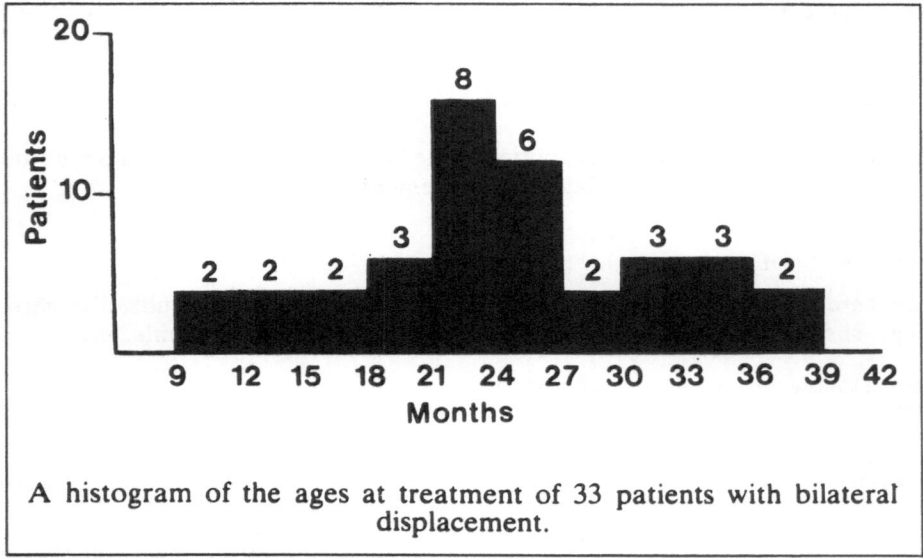

A histogram of the ages at treatment of 33 patients with bilateral displacement.

Fig. 4.33. Histograms showing age at diagnosis in unilateral and bilateral displacement

BILATERAL DISPLACEMENT

There were 33 patients with 66 hips which were displaced. Comparing these with the unilateral displacements shows that the results of the unilaterally dislocated hips was rather better than those with bilateral dislocation, with 80% acceptable as against 74%, but the rate of unacceptable hips was twice as great among the bilateral cases.

SECONDARY OPERATIONS

Because of recurring deformity secondary osteotomies were carried out in 20 hips. As might be expected, the results were inferior to those of primary treatment; only 60% were considered acceptable. The impression gained was that the results would have been improved if operation had not been delayed too long in the forlorn hope that it could be avoided. It was clear that if once a hip has demonstrably started to deteriorate it will worsen unless something is done to stop it. The deterioration does not stop on its own.

ROTATION OSTEOTOMY WITH VARUS

The one variant from the routine treatment which was obviously successful was the combination of a small amount of varus with the rotation at the osteotomy. Although only 17 of these had been done long enough ago to be included in the series the results were in every way superior to those in which rotation alone was done, 90% being acceptable at the time of examination. But not only were the later results better; the immediate results were also better. The child walks better, with the foot to the front, right from the start.

Progress after Treatment

From the examination of a series of radiographs (Figs. 5.10–5.15) it is clear that if the examination is carried out at different times during the progress of development different assessments of the results may be made. In an attempt to estimate the improvement or deterioration of hips over the years a series of hips was reviewed at 5, 10, 15 and 20 or more years. The results of this investigation are seen in Table 4.3. It can be seen that there was an apparent improvement between 5 and 10 years, presumably because ossification was improving. There was then an appreciable fall in the number which were acceptable and a bigger rise in the number unacceptable, followed by a flattening-out of the deterioration later.

Table 4.3. Results at 5-yearly intervals

	Acceptable	Uncertain	Unacceptable
At 5 years	65%	25%	10%
At 10 years	80%	12%	8%
At 15 years	73%	13%	13%
At 20 years	74%	9%	17%

While it was always clear that there would be progressive deterioration, among those that were less than good there was also a suggestion that in some of those hips in which the acetabular development was acceptable there was some slight deterioration which would need watching.

SEQUELAE

Because of the degenerative changes previously suspected a further review was carried out 5½ years later (Somerville 1980). We reviewed 107 hips which had been followed up for 15–30 years and in which it was considered that at some time during their development the acetabular development had been satisfactory. The distribution is shown in Table 4.4.

Table 4.4. Distribution of 107 treated hips

Initial condition	No. of hips
Dislocations	
Unilateral	65
Bilateral	26
Subluxations	
Unilateral	14
Bilateral	2
	107

In 65 patients the dislocations were unilateral and in 13 they were bilateral. Deterioration was assessed on narrowing of the joint space with thinning of the articular cartilage, subchondral sclerosis, and marginal lipping.

Among the 16 hips which had initially been subluxated there did not appear to have been any deterioration. Among the 91 hips which had been dislocated there was some radiologically obvious change in 19. In 11 the changes were obvious and in eight they were minimal. In the unilateral dislocations 11 of the 65 hips showed some change, obvious (Fig. 4.34) in seven and minimal (Fig. 4.35) in four. In the bilateral

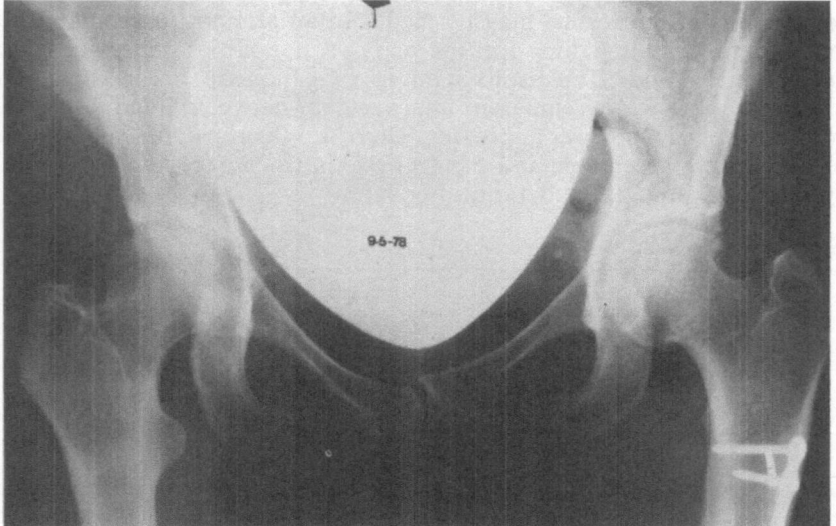

Fig. 4.34. Obvious degenerative changes in the left hip of a patient aged 32 years, who was treated for a dislocation 30 years previously

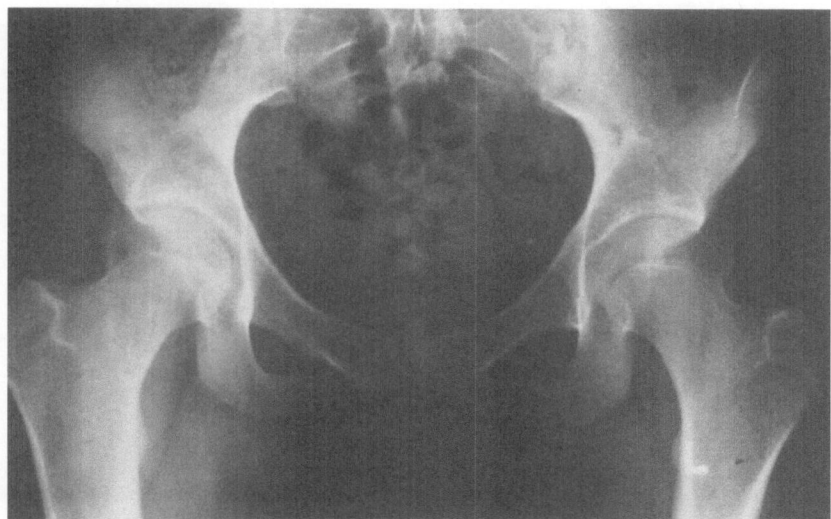

Fig. 4.35. The left hip, although well developed, is showing early evidence of thinning of the articular cartilage

dislocations 8 of the 26 hips showed changes, obvious (Fig. 4.36) in four and minimal (Fig. 4.37) in four.

CE ANGLE

The CE angle was taken as the measurement of acetabular development. To ascertain what the CE angle should have been following treatment the angle in the

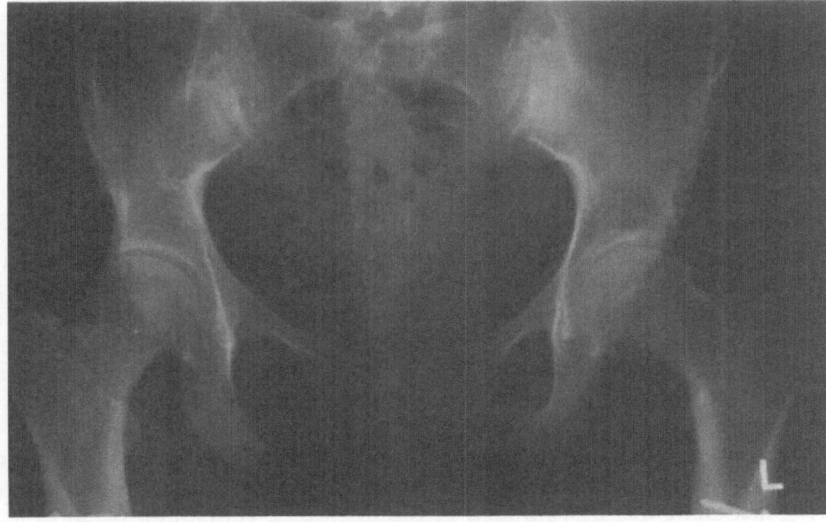

Fig. 4.36. Following the treatment of severe bilateral dislocations both hips have developed well, but 27 years later both are showing some evidence of deterioration

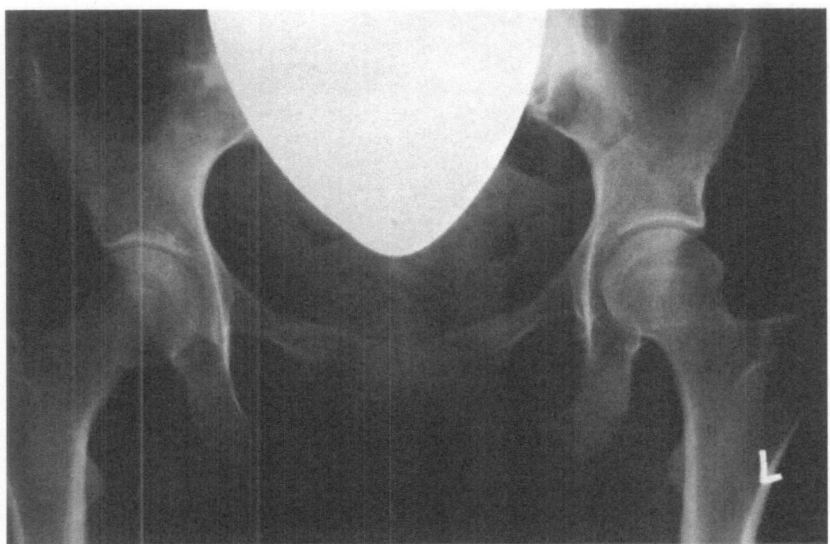

Fig. 4.37. Bilateral dislocations treated 18 years previously have developed excellently, but in the right hip there is some thinning of the articular cartilage

untreated hip was taken as a model in those with unilateral dislocation. This made it possible to divide the 65 patients into three groups. In group I the CE angle was the same in both hips. In group II the CE angle was greater in the untreated than in the treated hip, and in group III the CE angle was greater in the treated than in the normal hip. The distribution is seen in Table 4.5.

Table 4.5. CE angle following treatment for dislocation of the hip

Group	No. of patients	No. with changes	
		Obvious	Minimal
I	21	0	2
II	22	2	2
III	22	5	2

In group I only minimal changes were seen in two hips. In group II obvious wear was seen in two hips, and in one of them this was severe. In one the development was satisfactory until the age of 11 (Fig. 4.38). At 12 years (Fig. 4.39) it was only with hindsight that the minimal displacement could be seen. Unfortunately the child was not seen for 7 years and by then the displacement was marked and beyond repair (Fig. 4.40). The only known clinical abnormality was a recurrence of anteversion, which unfortunately had been ignored. If this had been corrected there is a possibility that the subsequent changes might have been prevented.

A similar subluxation taking place in the same age group is seen in Fig. 4.41. This hip had always been normal and there had never been anything wrong with it. Displacement was first noticed at the age of 12 years, and because no action was taken developed into a severe subluxation with marked changes in the acetabulum (Fig. 4.42), which necessitated a pelvic and femoral osteotomy at the same time. This

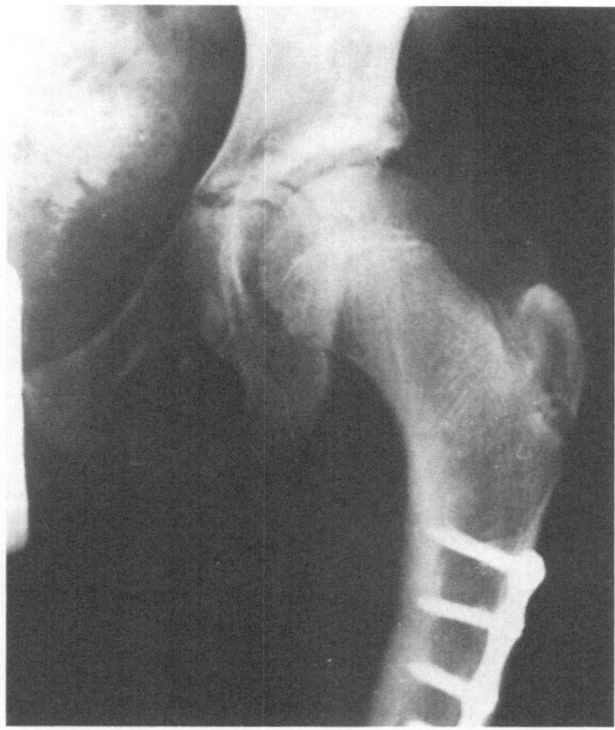

Fig. 4.38. This hip was treated for dislocation at the age of 2 years. At the age of 11 the appearance suggests that development has been excellent

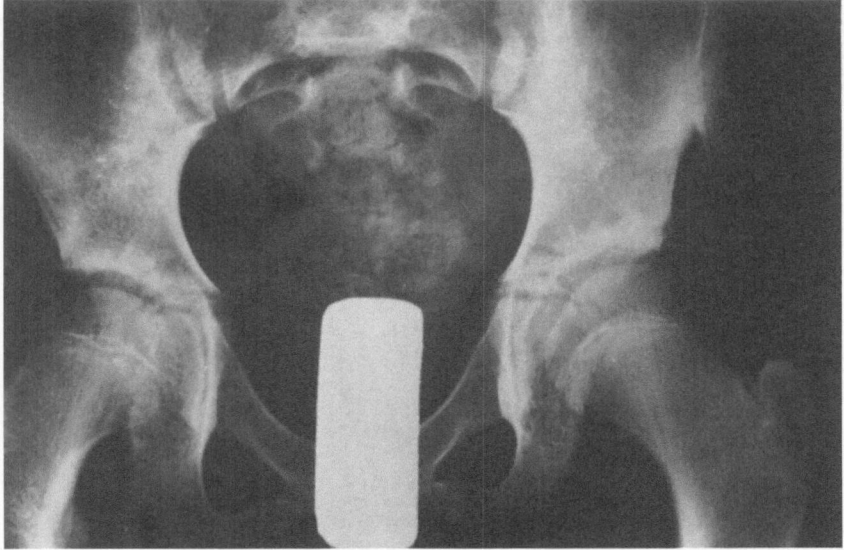

Fig. 4.39. The same hip as shown in Fig. 4.38 seen 1 year later. The child herself was not seen and the x-ray appearance was considered to be satisfactory. With hindsight minimal displacement can be seen

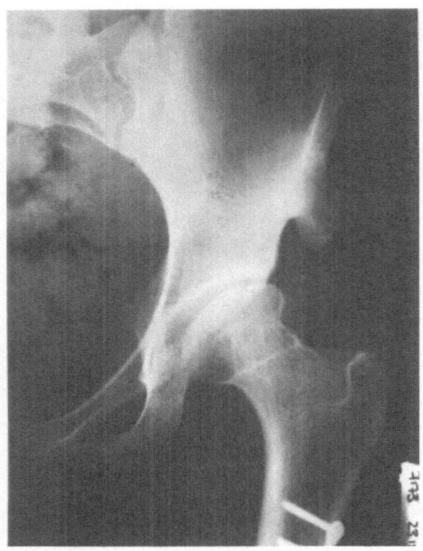

Fig. 4.40. Six years after the examination illustrated in Fig. 4.39 there are marked changes, which are irreversible

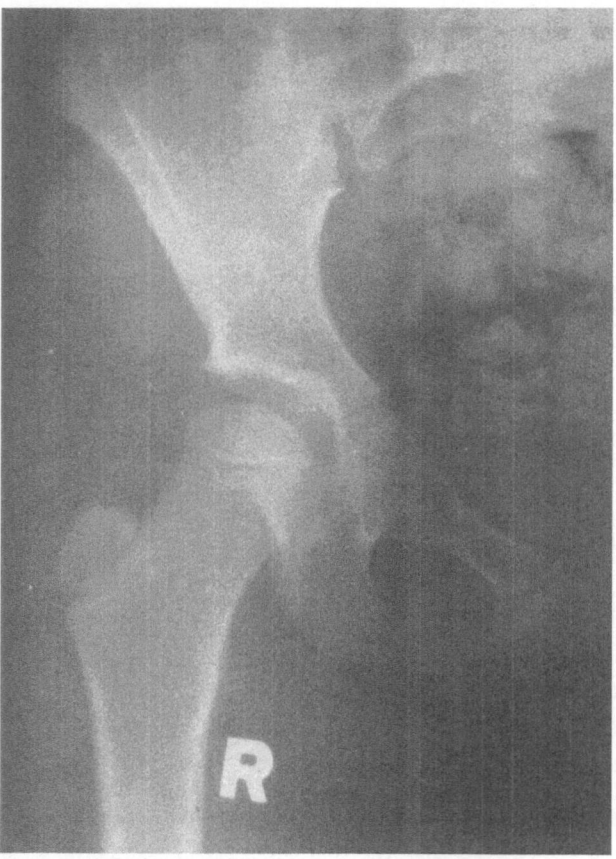

Fig. 4.41. A hip which has developed normally up to the age of 11 years

displacement was also associated with persistent foetal alignment and was symptom-free throughout. The second case showing wear in group II was the only known case in which damage was done to the hyaline cartilaginous lip of the acetabulum when the limbus was being excised. When the limbus was examined histologically a small sliver of cartilage was found. The hip continued to develop well (Fig. 4.43) until the age of 22 years, when minor changes were noted (Fig. 4.44). The deterioration progressed rapidly until a severe arthritis had developed (Fig. 4.45).

In group III seven of the 22 hips showed evidence of wear. In five they were obvious and in two minimal, suggesting that the depth of the acetabulum is an important factor in the longer-term result but not always in the way that might have been expected. It appears that a too-deep acetabulum may be more to be feared than one which is too shallow, provided that the hip with the shallow acetabulum is stable (Fig. 4.46). Obviously it is important to examine the factors that influence the depth of the acetabulum during growth.

The mechanics of the joint play a large part in the development. Anteversion and valgus cause the acetabulum to be shallow and to develop less well, whereas it seems that the absence of anteversion combined with a slight excess of varus will cause it to develop better and, as appears from this review, sometimes too deeply. In group III there were five hips in which this phenomenon was seen. In three of these hips the CE angle was over 40°. In all there was a slight increase in the angle of varus (Fig. 4.34) and possibly a very slight degree of retroversion. In this position the head of the femur is directed into the bare area of the acetabulum. This is a common finding in cases of protrussio acetabuli. While a minor degree of excess varus will cause the acetabulum to develop too deeply, a more marked degree, while having other disadvantages, will not (Fig. 4.47). It seems that the angle must be just right.

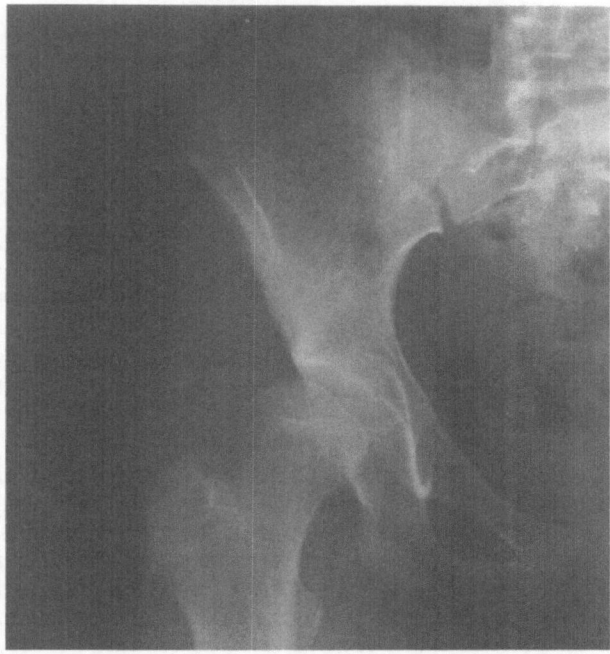

Fig. 4.42. Same hip as in Fig. 4.41. During the intervening 3 years increasing displacement has taken place

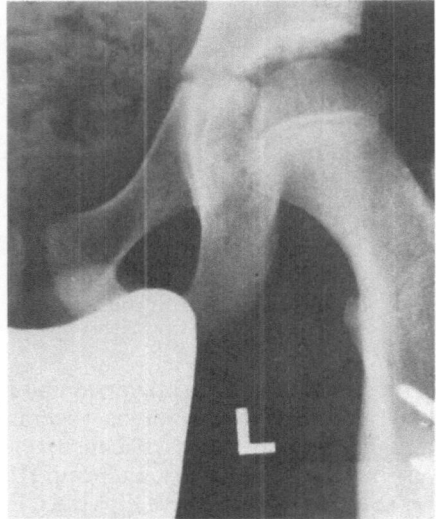

Fig. 4.43. At the age of 15 this hip is seen to
have developed well

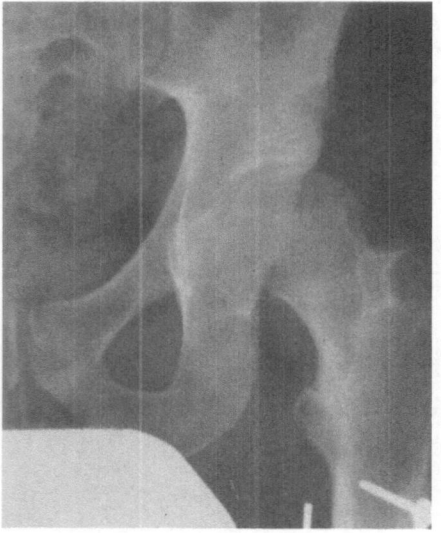

Fig. 4.44. At the age of 22 years there is a
suggestion that the joint illustrated in Fig. 4.43 is
becoming narrow

In spite of this a little varus in excess early on may be of value, and since the
introduction of this routinely it seems that the results have improved. This is well
illustrated in the following case. A child was treated for severe dislocations. At the
age of 4½ years, although the hips were well reduced, a severe coxa valga developed
(Fig. 4.48). There had been no recurrence of anteversion. Varus osteotomies were
carried out but the amount of varus on the right was rather more than on the left,
which looked rather the better of the two. Both hips developed normally for some
years (Fig. 4.49), but it later became apparent that while the hip on the right
continued to develop well, the one on the left progressively deteriorated (Fig. 4.50).

It has been suggested that the cause of central degeneration is coxa vara, combined
perhaps with slight retroversion, so it must be very unusual for such changes to
develop in the presence of coxa valga. Nevertheless, there was one patient who was

treated for severe bilateral dislocations who developed severe coxa valga (Fig. 4.51). Because this did not interfere with the development of the acetabula it was not corrected. It can be seen that there is excellent development of the acetabula but central degeneration is becoming apparent in both hips, with thinning of the articular cartilage, which must have been caused by some mechanism other than that already described.

It is possible that when the acetabulum is exceptionally well developed, either naturally or as the result of operation, the roof may slope upwards and medially from the rim. In this circumstance every time weight is taken on the leg the femoral head will be displaced medially against the medial wall of the acetabulum, gradually causing damage to the articular cartilage in this area.

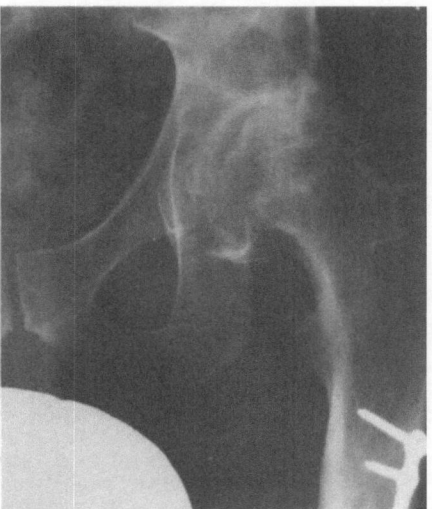

Fig. 4.45. At the age of 27 the hip shown in Figs. 4.43 and 4.44 is grossly arthritic

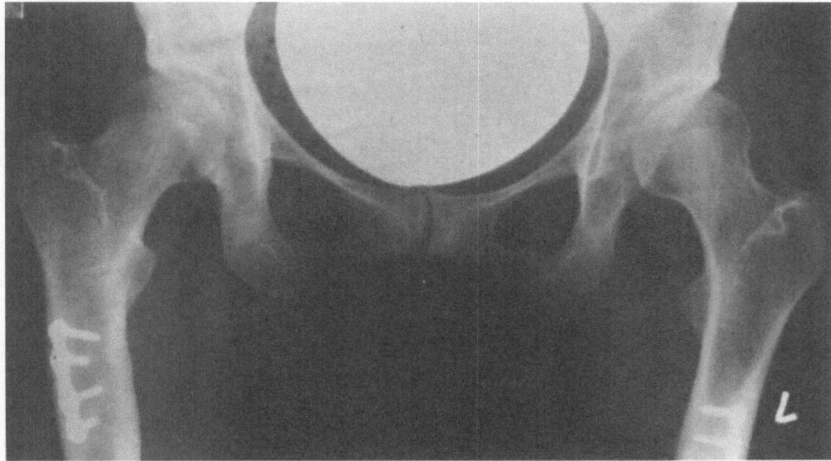

Fig. 4.46. This child had a subluxation of the right hip and a dislocation of the left, treated at the age of 20 months. Twenty-three years later the left hip shows evidence of a minor degree of subluxation but no evidence of wear, because it is stable

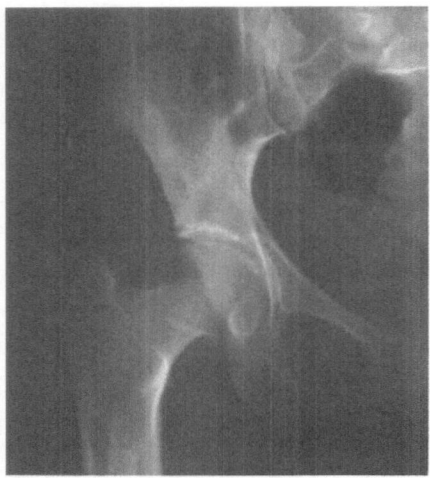

Fig. 4.47. A more excessive degree of varus has led to the development of a good acetabulum and there is no suggestion of thinning of the articular cartilage

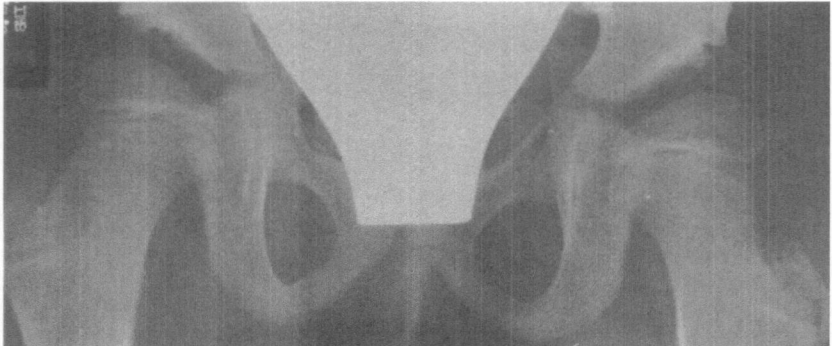

Fig. 4.48. By 2½ years after the treatment of severe bilateral dislocations a marked coxa valga has developed, which is interfering with development

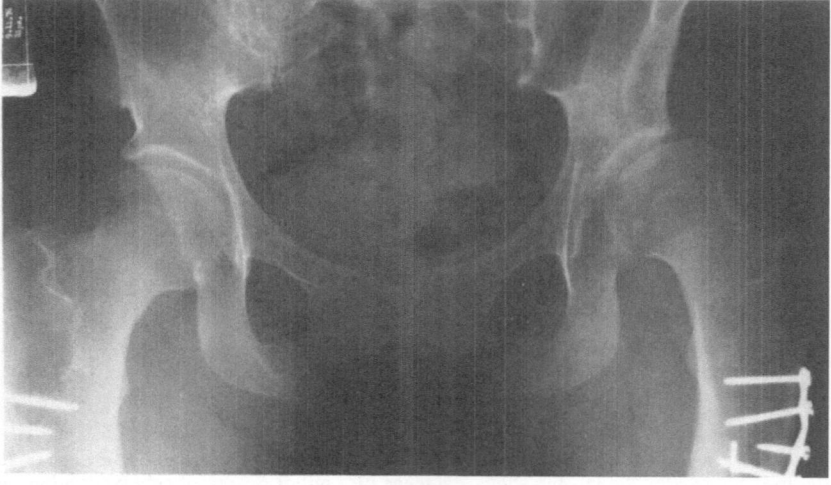

Fig. 4.49. Same patient as in Fig. 4.47. Four years later both hips are developing well

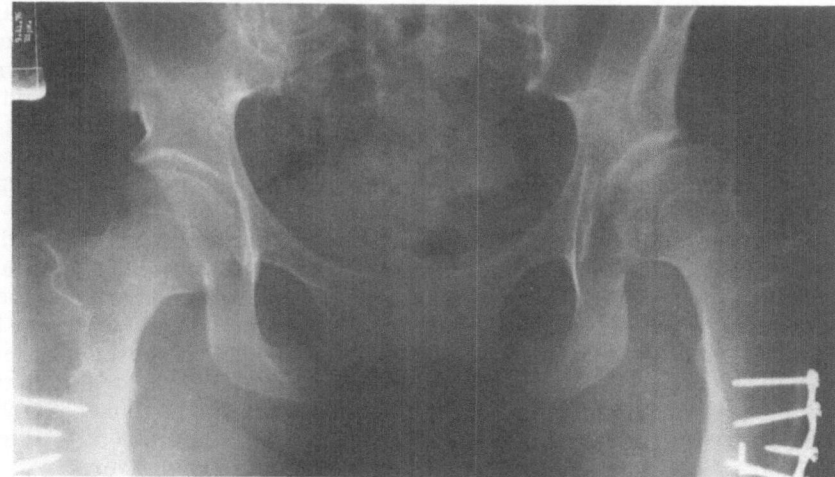

Fig. 4.50. At the age of 20 it is clear that in the same patient as in Figs. 4.48 and 4.49 the right hip, where there was rather more varus, has developed well but the left hip is deteriorating

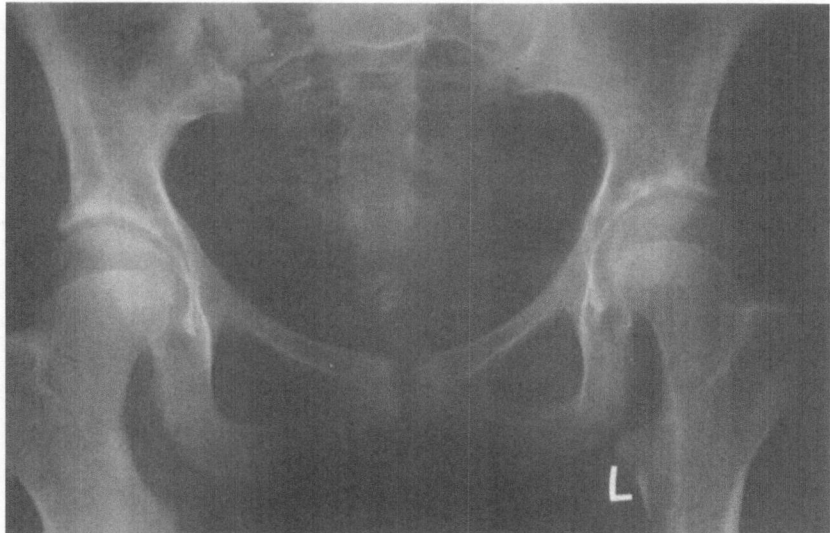

Fig. 4.51. Well-marked coxa valga has developed following the treatment of severe bilateral dislocations. This did not affect the development of the acetabula, which are rather over-developed. At the age of 19 there is obvious thinning of the articular cartilage medially

DISCUSSION

Sir Harry Platt (1953), in an editorial, said that we should not be too perfectionist in our treatment of the congenitally dislocated hip, because even a good result could hardly be expected to last for more than 25 years. With present knowledge this view seems to be a little pessimistic. But it does raise some very interesting points. Wynne-Davies (1970) has stated that in normal hips the CE angle increases with age, presumably due to thinning of the articular cartilage. The results obtained in the series just quoted suggest that the acetabulum which becomes too deep can give rise to trouble. We know only too well how many hips which at one time were probably normal have reached a stage of arthritis by the age of 50 when consideration is being given to total prosthetic replacement, either because of the development of subluxation or because the acetabulum has become too deep. If this is the natural history of the normal hip in many cases, how much more is it likely to occur in a hip which was initially dislocated for 2 years?

What sort of hip will last the longest? It seems that one which is exactly right may last a life-time but one which is only very slightly different will in due course become either too deep or too shallow, with inevitable deterioration. It seems, then, that if as a result of treatment we have failed to produce perfection and we have a hip which is stable but a little too shallow, we are unlikely to delay the onset of degeneration by making it deeper. We may in fact precipitate the arthritis we are attempting to delay for the sake of a slightly more acceptable radiological appearance. All of this is pure conjecture with no proof, only suspicion (Figs. 5.57, 5.58 and 5.59). Unfortunately it will take more than one orthopaedic life-time to find an answer.

REFERENCES

Mitchel GP (1963) Arthrography in congenital dislocation of the hip. J Bone Joint Surg [Br] 44:219
Platt Sir Harry (1953) Congenital dislocation of the hip. (Editorial) J Bone Joint Surg [Br] 35:339
Scott JC (1953) Frame reduction in congenital dislocation of the hip. J Bone Joint Surg [Br] 35:372
Severin E (1941) Contribution to the knowledge of congenital dislocation of the hip joints. Late results of closed reduction and arthrographic studies of recent cases. Acta Chir Scand 84 [Suppl 63]:1
Severin E (1950) Congenital dislocation of the hip. Development of the joint after closed reduction. J Bone Joint Surg [Am] 32:507
Somerville EW (1953) Open reduction in congenital dislocation of the hip. J Bone Joint Surg [Br] 35:363
Somerville EW (1978) A long term follow-up of congenital dislocation of the hip. J Bone Joint Surg [Br] 60:25
Somerville EW (1980) Congenital dislocation of the hip. The fate of the well-developed acetabulum. Isr J Med Sci 16/4:338
Somerville EW, Scott JC (1957) The direct approach to congenital dislocation of the hip. J Bone Joint Surg [Br] 39:623
Wynne-Davies R (1970) Acetabular dysplasia and familial joint laxity. J Bone Joint Surg [Br] 52:704

5 Development of the Hip

The most important phase in the treatment of the congenitally dislocated hip is the follow-up. Treatment is not complete when the child leaves hospital. The hip has a great many years in which to grow, and the way in which it grows is all-important.

A number of factors affect the way in which a bone develops. When initially formed in cartilage it has a definite shape, which will be modified by the stresses to which it is subjected, by the distribution of the blood supply, and most of all by the growth plate (Trueta 1957). Anything that affects any one of these will cause the bone to grow in a different way. This will modify its mechanics and also the development of any joint with which it is involved.

After hospital treatment is completed it is quite impossible to say whether any of these factors will play a part in the future development of the hip. If the situation has been explained beforehand to the parents they will be more ready to accept that further operation may prove necessary to prevent deterioration of the hip in their apparently normal child.

NORMAL

At the time of birth almost the whole of the upper end of the femur is composed of cartilage. Ossification progresses upwards from the growth centre in the shaft to form the metaphysis, which extends from the medial side of the neck to the lateral side of the greater trochanter. Harris's line gives a clear indication of the way in which the upper end of the femur grows from this metaphysis (Fig. 3.5). The capital ossific nucleus is first seen at about the sixth month, but the ossific nucleus of the greater trochanter is not seen until about the fifth year.

Similarly, at the time of birth the acetabulum is very poorly ossified (Fig. 5.1), but ossification takes place rapidly, so that by the age of 8 months a well-recognised socket can be seen (Fig. 5.2). Nevertheless it will be a further 2 or 3 years before it becomes fully defined (Figs. 5.3–5.5).

Normal Development of the Abnormal Hip

AFTER EARLY TREATMENT

Following successful treatment of a dislocated or dislocatable hip diagnosed at birth, ossification takes place as in the normal hip. There is little, if any, delay in the appearance of the ossific nucleus, and ossification of the acetabulum is within normal limits. Delay in ossification compared with the normal side suggests that some minor degree of instability still persists. Such an appearance need not cause alarm and is not

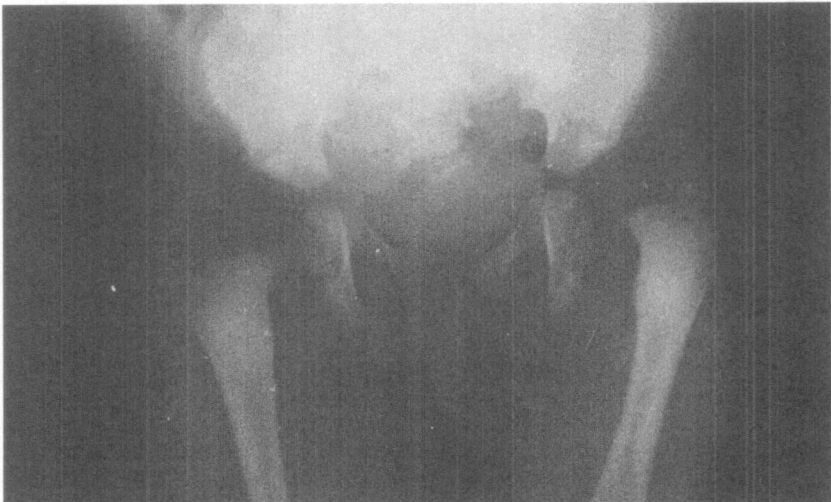

Fig. 5.1. The right hip is normal, the left displaced. There is nothing to choose between the ossification of the two at the time of birth

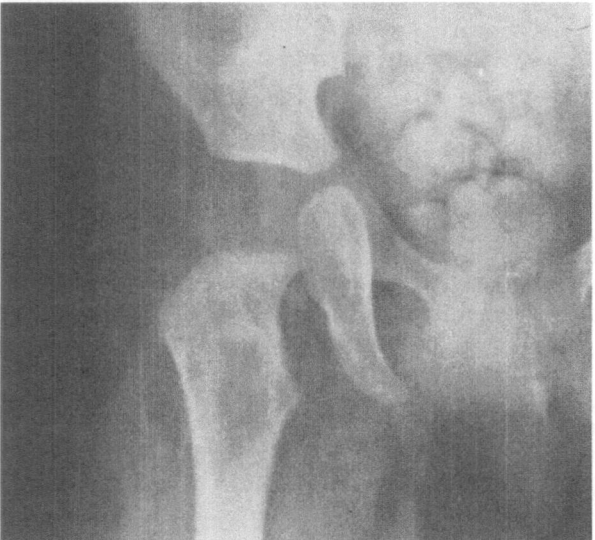

Fig. 5.2. The normal hip shown in Fig. 5.1, at the age of 8 months. The ossification of the acetabulum has improved and the nucleus in the femoral head is visible

an indication for resumption of splintage. Such hips will develop normally over 1 or 2 years, as has been noted in Chapter 2. The appearance of obvious subluxation in the presence of normal ossification (Fig. 5.6) is usually of little consequence and needs no treatment. Such hips will develop normally over a number of years (Figs. 5.7 and 5.8), but they should be monitored at yearly intervals until growth is complete. Hips in which there is both delayed ossification and obvious subluxation are fortunately uncommon, but they need much more careful watching and may well require correction by femoral osteotomy, though there is no hurry about doing this.

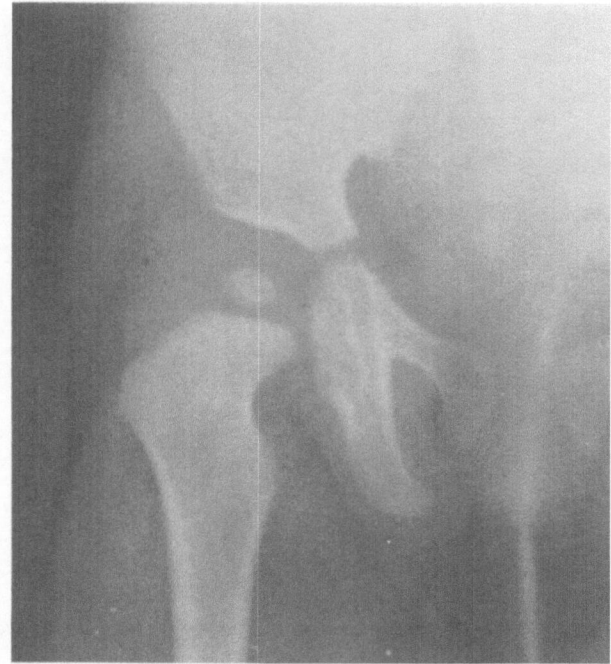

Fig. 5.3. The same hip as shown in Figs. 5.1 and 5.2, at the age of 16 months. Ossification in the head is good but the ossification in the acetabulum is still incomplete

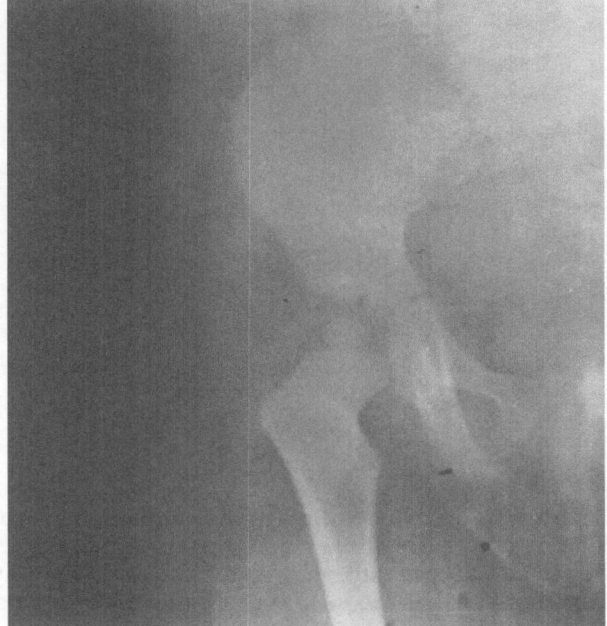

Fig. 5.4. At 2 years ossification in the acetabulum is still incomplete

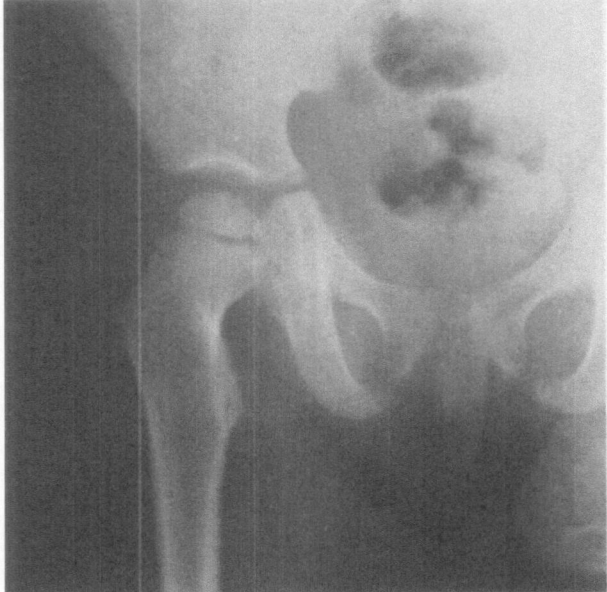

Fig. 5.5. It is not until the age of 3½ years that ossification in the acetabulum is seen to be complete

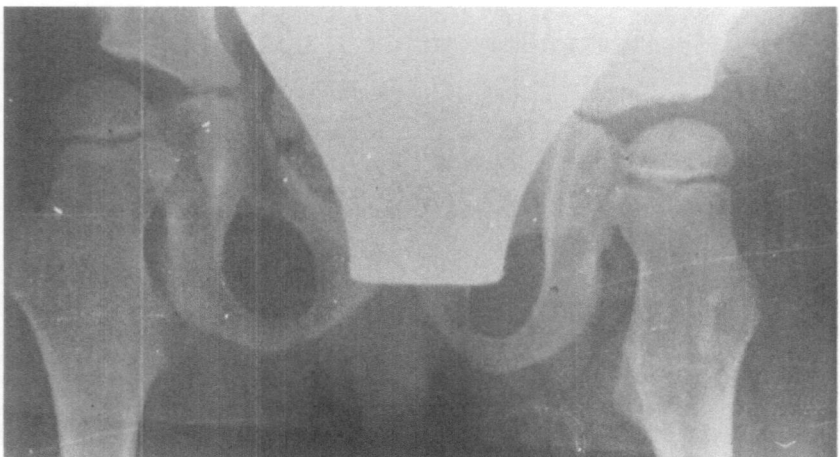

Fig. 5.6. Hips of a child aged 2½ years who has not received any treatment. There is coxa valga and some subluxation on both sides. Ossification is normal

AFTER-TREATMENT OF ESTABLISHED DISPLACEMENT

The follow-up of patients with established displacement should be arranged at a special clinic and a visual record kept to demonstrate progress. A convenient way of doing this is to mount photographs of the radiographs on a large sheet, so that a consecutive series can be seen at a glance and a comparison made. The importance of this is that it is not possible to determine the progress of a hip for better or for worse from a single radiograph; it can be done only from a series (Fig. 5.9).

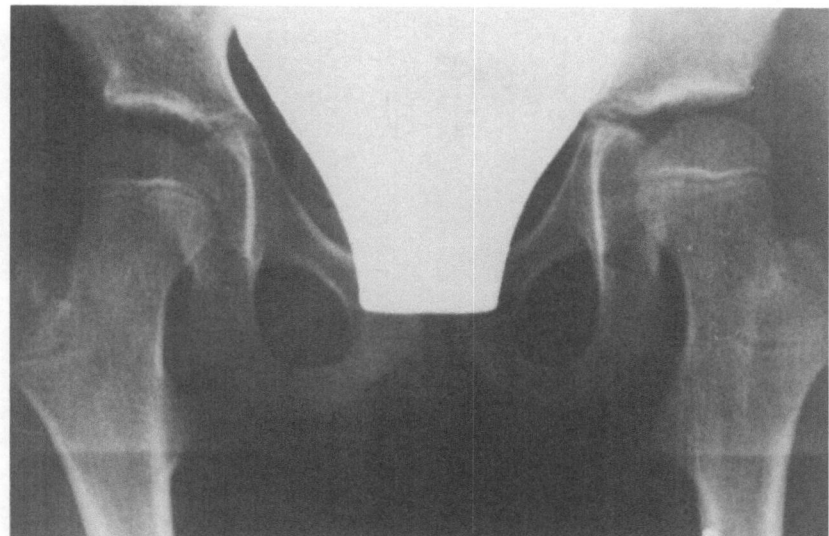

Fig. 5.7. At the age of 6 there is appreciable improvement in the hips shown in Fig. 5.6

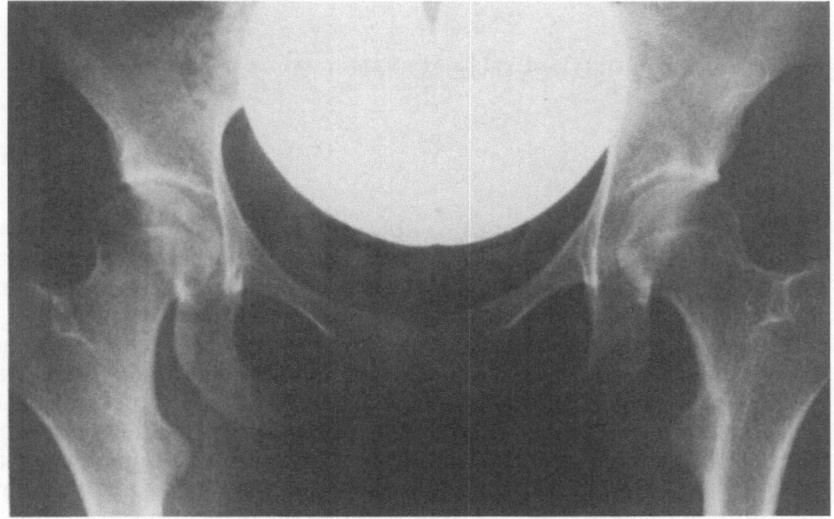

Fig. 5.8. At the age of 16 both hips shown in Figs. 5.6 and 5.7 are normal, with normal neck-shaft angles and Shenton's lines intact

At the head of each sheet is recorded the name and address, date of birth, age at diagnosis, age at the commencement of walking, family history and if possible particulars of birth. The first six radiographs record the stages of treatment; the seventh is taken 3 months after discharge, the eighth 6 months later; and subsequent ones record the position at yearly intervals. The date is recorded beneath each radiograph together with, if relevant, what it shows; between the radiographs treatment undertaken and the date of it are recorded.

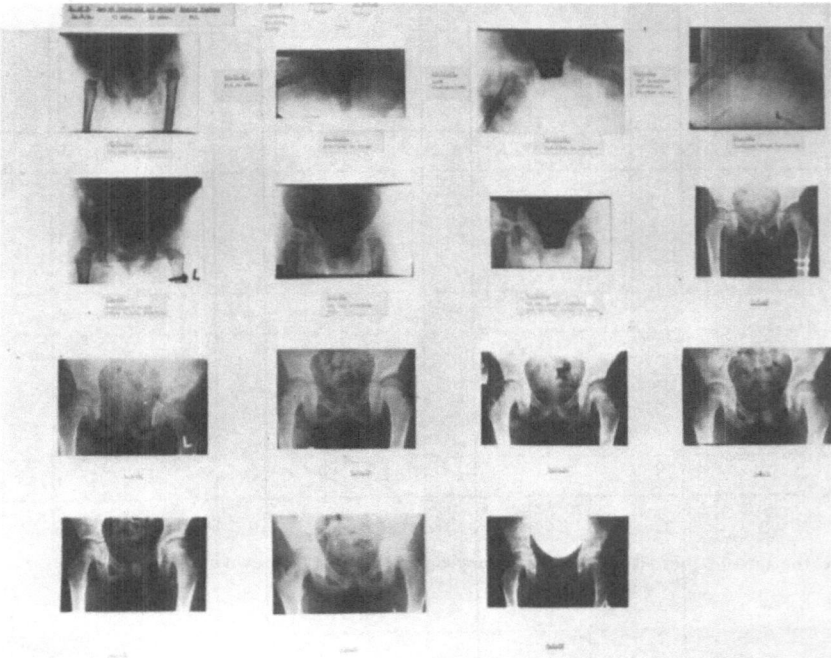

Fig. 5.9. Visual record card used for following up all cases of congenital dislocation of the hip

When established subluxation or dislocation has been successfully treated with the restoration of concentric movement, ossification of the capital ossific nucleus will take place rapidly, but ossification of the acetabulum may be slow and in some cases may take many years to be completed (Figs. 5.10–5.15).

The development of the ossific nucleus of the head of the femur may not always be quite straightforward. In Chapter 3 mention has been made of the ways in which ossification may be affected by damage to the blood supply due to the dislocation and occurring before treatment is undertaken. It is the medial side of the ossific nucleus that is late to appear and slow to develop, so that for some time during the development it is only the lateral part of the nucleus that is visible, and this may be smaller than normal because of the instability. When the displacement is reduced the upper end of the femur is stimulated to grow: it will grow rapidly and may even grow larger than the normal side. But it is still only one half of the nucleus that can grow, and this may lead to considerable disproportion between the sides of the head. This disproportion may persist without presenting any problem, but as discussed later it may cause overgrowth and an increase in valgus to a point where redisplacement may occur.

Ossification of the acetabulum may proceed in various ways. Sometimes it is orderly, as in a normal joint, the ossification spreading throughout the cartilaginous roof of the acetabulum. Occasionally bone may be laid down in layers like an onion (Fig. 5.16). More often an ossific nucleus will appear in the acetabular roof, with which it will ultimately fuse (Figs. 5.17 and 5.18); most commonly multiple nuclei

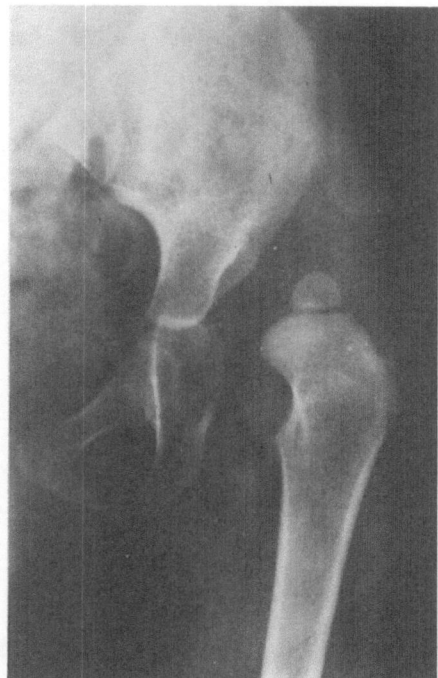

Fig. 5.10. Dislocated hip in a child aged 2 years.
There is very poor ossification in the acetabular roof
and in the head

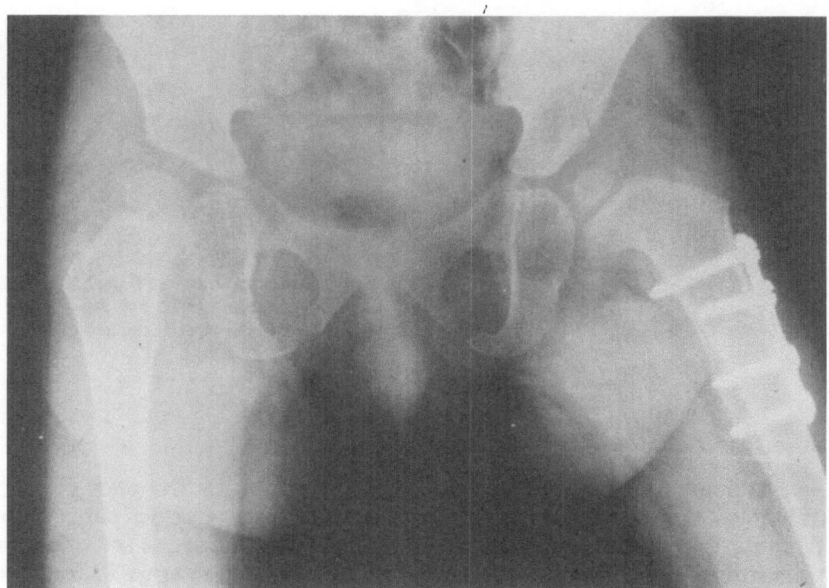

Fig. 5.11. The same hip as in Fig. 5.10 at completion of treatment, when unrestricted mobilisation was
started

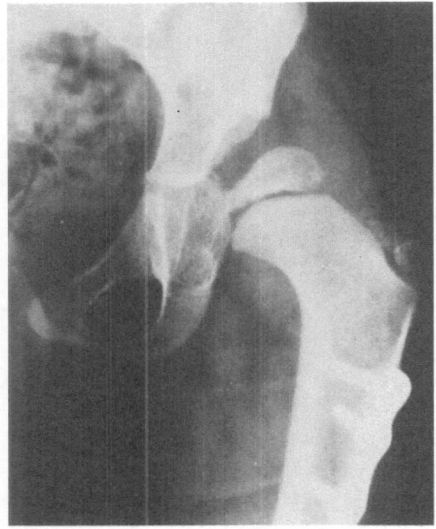

Fig. 5.12. One year later ossification in the hip shown in Figs. 5.10 and 5.11 is still very defective. The child is fully active

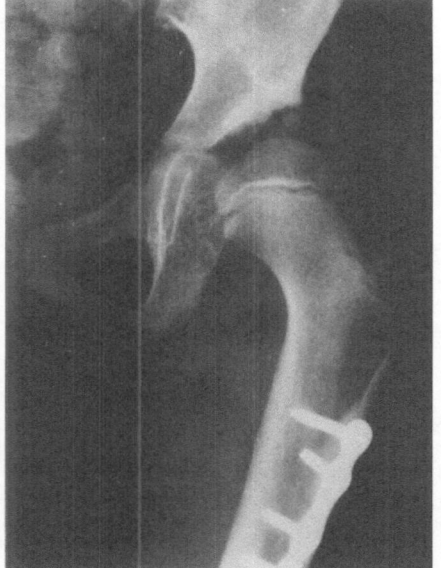

Fig. 5.13. Three-and-a-half years after treatment of the hip shown in Figs. 5.10–5.12 there is a marked improvement. An ossific nucleus can be seen in the roof of the acetabulum

will appear, and with time, fuse together and with the roof (Figs. 5.13–5.15). Whatever the process of the ossification, the appearance will suggest roughness and irregularity. This is apparent and not real, and is evidence of active growth which will persist until consolidation is completed between the ages of 12 and 14 years (Figs. 5.14 and 5.15). None of these appearances need cause concern; nor are they a reason for further treatment, so long as radiographs taken at yearly intervals show a progressive improvement.

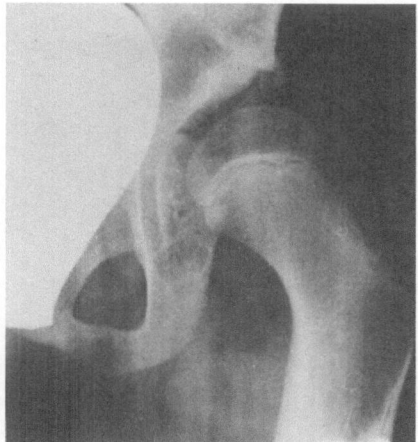

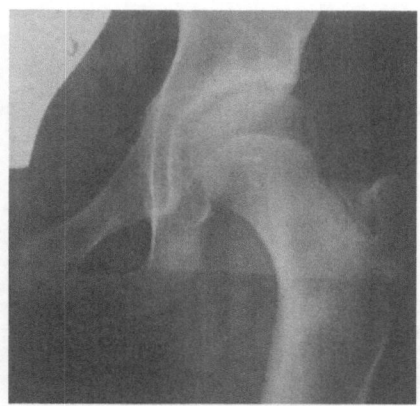

Fig. 5.15. At the age of 18 the hip shown in Figs. 5.10–5.14 is normal

Fig. 5.14. Further improvement in the hip shown in Figs. 5.10–5.13 is visible 2 years later

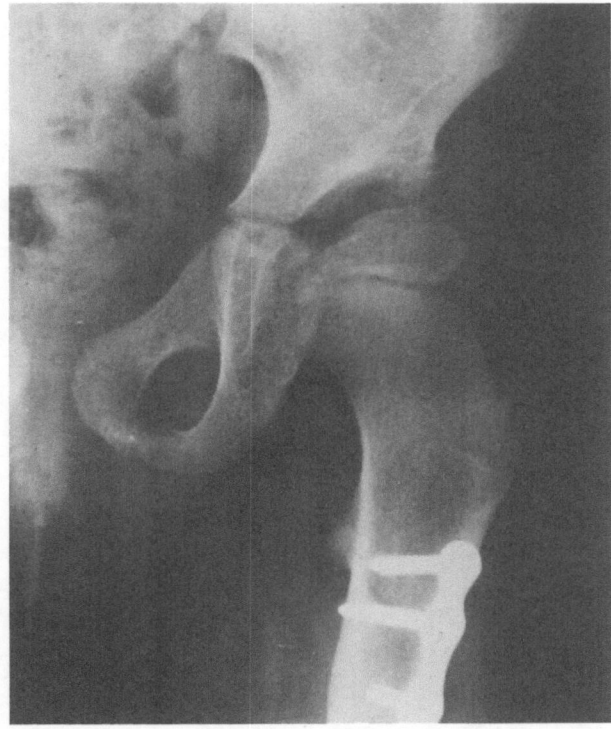

Fig. 5.16. The way in which the acetabulum has extended out over the head of the femur can be seen from the line which still indicates the outer limit of the ossification of the pelvis as it was at the time of treatment

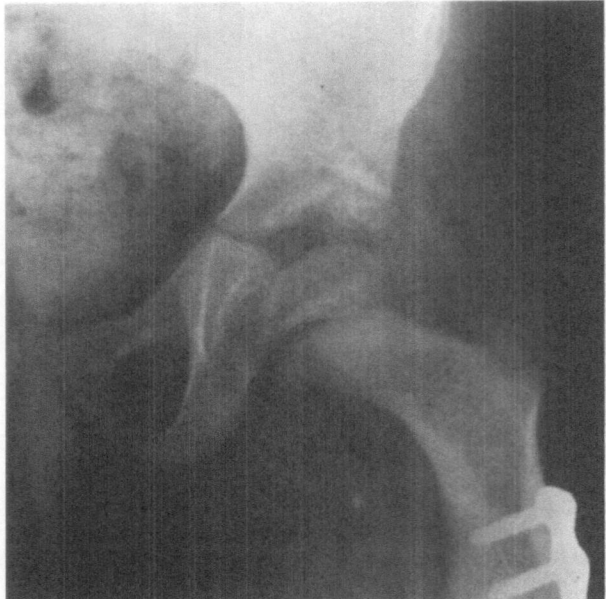

Fig. 5.17. A more common way in which ossification takes place is by the development of a nucleus in the cartilaginous roof

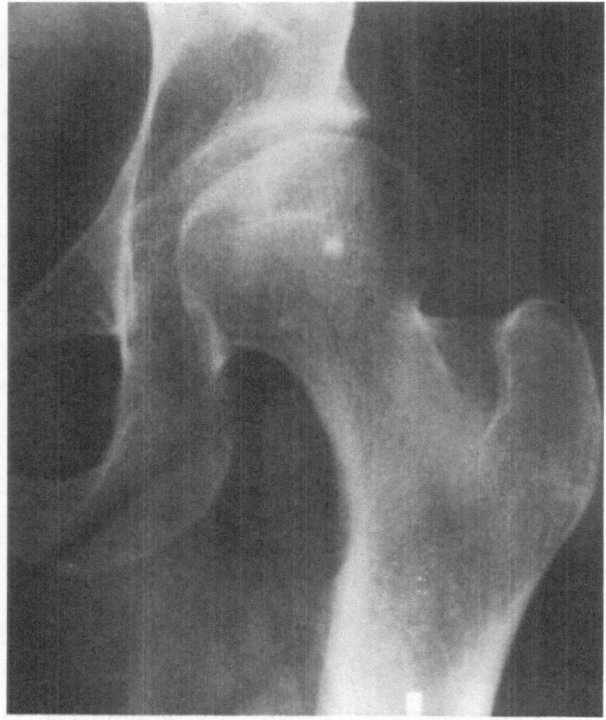

Fig. 5.18. The nucleus shown in Fig. 5.17 fuses with the main ossification

Abnormal Development of the Abnormal Hip

Deterioration in the ossification of the hip is evidence that there is an eccentric type of movement in the joint. This may have been present from the time of treatment and may be due to some technical failure; or it may have developed some years later as the result of a progressive recurrence of bone deformity. Occasionally, as will be seen, deterioration may be seen in a hip which has been normal at birth and for some years afterwards.

There can be few surgeons who treat congenital dislocation of the hip who have not had the unhappy experience of seeing a hip, which appeared to be satisfactory 3 years after treatment, not quite so good at 5 years, and an obvious failure at 8. The appearance of such a hip at first sight suggests that it is the acetabulum which is at fault. If a ball-and-socket joint is failing it seems only natural that it should be the socket which fails rather than the ball, and therefore that it is the acetabulum which needs correction. A review of the evidence, however, suggests that the reverse is true, and that the acetabulum will recover spontaneously unless there is something which is actively preventing it from doing so (Somerville 1974; Harris et al. 1975).

It is known that in newborns 60%–70% of those hips that are found to be unstable at birth will have become stable by the end of the first week of life without any treatment and that those in which instability persists will, with very few exceptions, become normal within 3 months with a simple form of splintage. Such well-established evidence makes the likelihood of primary dysplasia remote. Even when there is an established deformity, there is a strong tendency for the acetabulum to develop normally in the right environment. A hip in which there is a definite subluxation at the age of 17 months (Fig. 5.19) can be converted into a normal hip by the correction of the faulty mechanics by means of a suitable high femoral osteotomy, as seen 23 years after correction in the case illustrated in Fig. 5.20. But this is the simplest of all established deformities to correct, and the rate of development is only slightly slower than that of the normal hip.

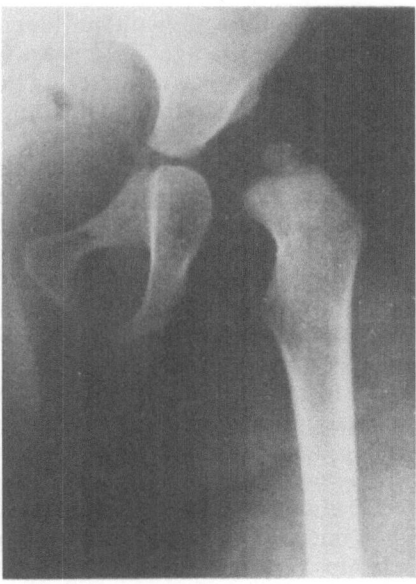

Fig. 5.19. A minor degree of displacement which was subsequently shown to be a subluxation. The sloping of the acetabular roof is only apparent, not real

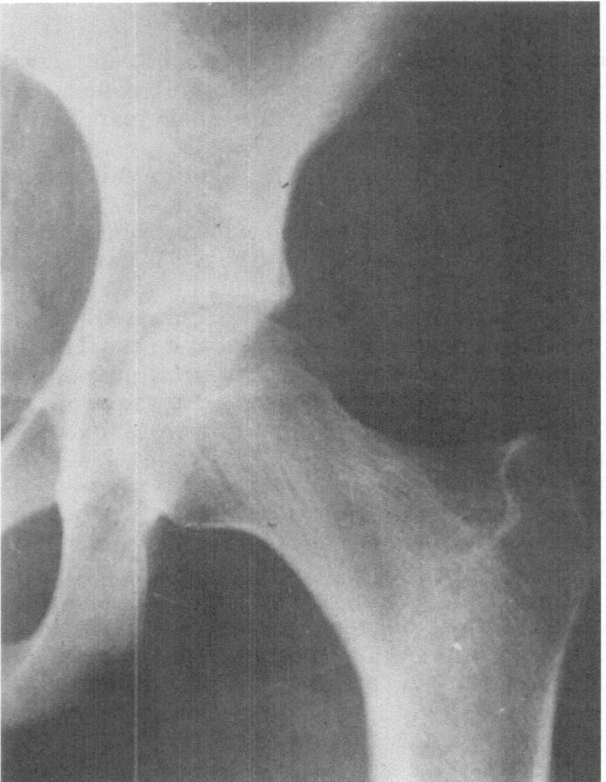

Fig. 5.20. The same hip as shown in Fig. 5.19, examined 23 years after high femoral rotation osteotomy

A rather more difficult problem is that presented by the child with bilateral dislocations at the age of 2½ years (Fig. 5.21). Correction of the mechanics of the joints, without in any way altering the shape of the acetabula, will allow the joints to develop normally, although the time taken to achieve normality will be longer (Fig. 5.22).

Much more difficulty is encountered with the hip which has undergone multiple treatments, all of which have been unsuccessful. Unilateral dislocation of the hip was diagnosed in a child at 1 year of age. Manipulative reduction was carried out, followed by 3 months in plaster in the frog position, at the end of which time it was found that the hip was still dislocated. Open reduction was attempted, followed by 9 months in plaster in the frog position. Because the hip was still dislocated a further open reduction was performed, followed by a high femoral osteotomy. At the time of admission to The Nuffield Orthopaedic Centre there was still displacement (Fig. 5.23). In abduction the head of the femur was seen to be hingeing on the lip of the acetabulum with no suggestion of reduction (Fig. 5.24). An extensive dissection of the hip, with replacement of the head centrally in the acetabulum, was followed by progressive improvement, without any structural change having been made in the acetabulum itself. Even after all this damage the acetabulum was still able to recover, when once it was given a chance to do so (Fig. 5.25).

In hips very severely damaged by treatment, where there can be no further hope of

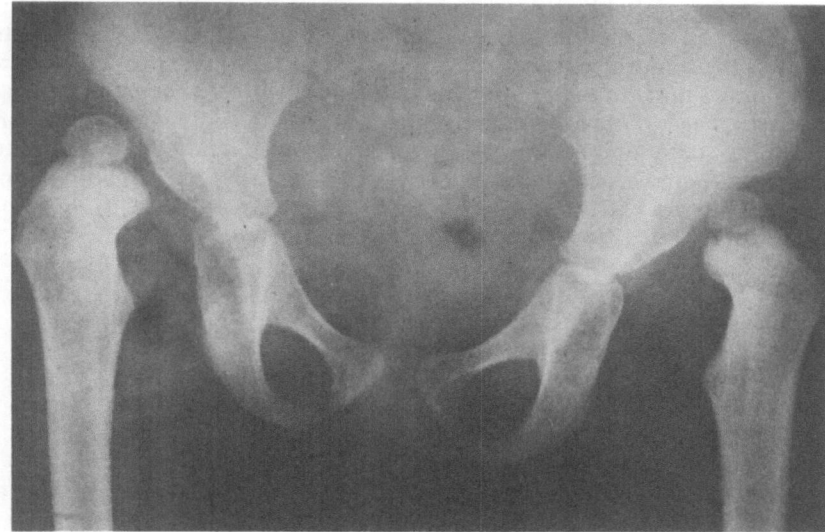

Fig. 5.21. Well-established bilateral dislocations of the hips in a child aged 2½ years

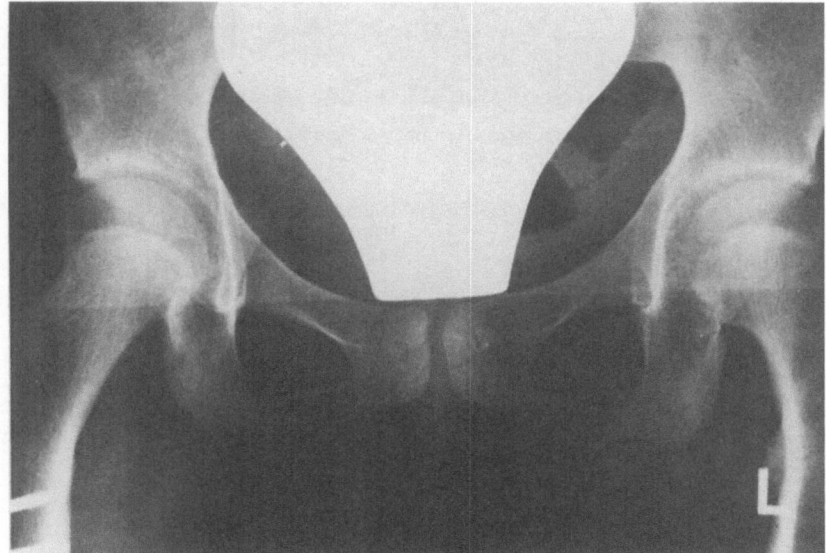

Fig. 5.22. The same hips as shown in Fig. 5.21, examined 23 years later

restoration to normality, the acetabulum will still make an extraordinary effort at regeneration once the deforming factors have been removed.

A child aged 2 years was found to have bilaterally dislocated hips. Attempted manipulative reductions were carried out and frog plasters applied with both hips dislocated, and these were retained for 3 months. Further manipulative reductions were carried out and the hips immobilised, this time in medial rotation but still in the displaced position. The right hip was abandoned, but on the left rotation osteotomy was performed without reduction. The position at the time of admission is shown in

Fig. 5.26. The right hip was treated along routine lines with frame reduction, excision of the limbus, and high femoral osteotomy. An open reduction with central replacement of the femoral head was performed on the left. The result 20 years later (Fig. 5.27) shows that the right hip has developed well, and even on the left, in spite of the severe damage to the growth plate and to the blood supply to the head of the femur, the hip is stable and a series of radiographs reveals no evidence of deterioration. Clinically there was an almost full range of flexion but limited abduction; there was no pain and the patient had no limp.

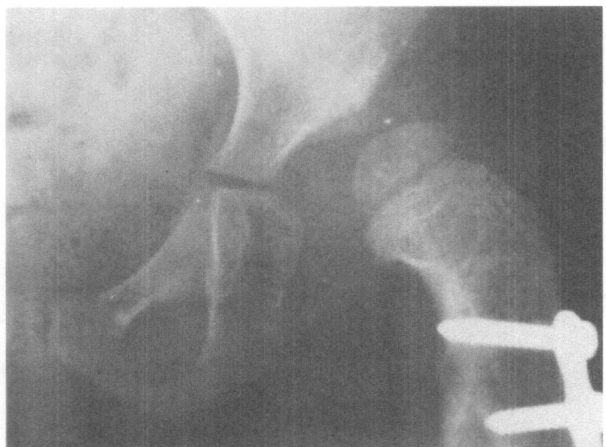

Fig. 5.23. Displacement is persistent after many attempts at reduction have failed

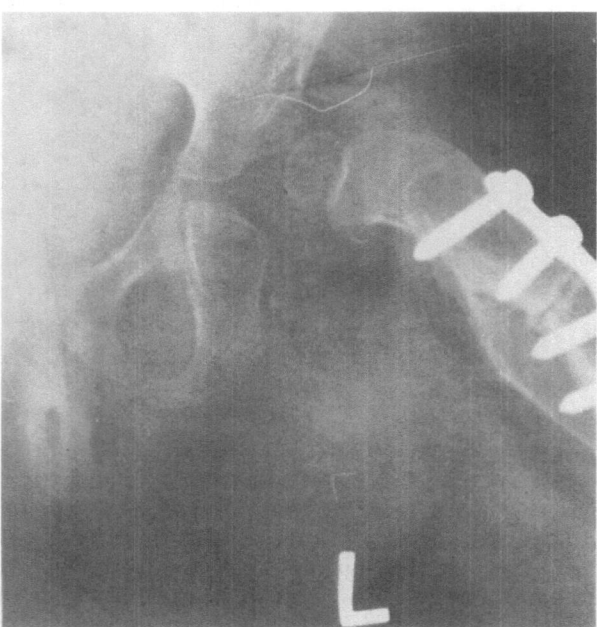

Fig. 5.24. In abduction the position is not improved. The head hinges on the lip of the acetabulum

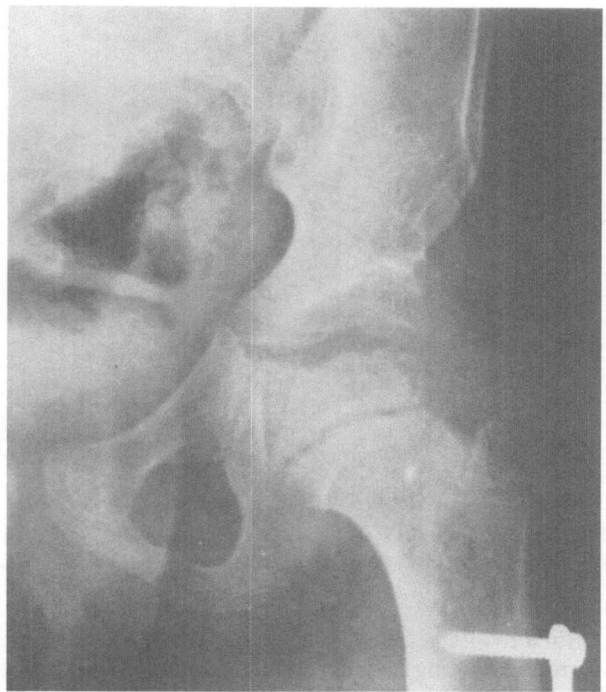

Fig. 5.25. Three years after attainment of concentric reduction of the hip shown in Figs. 5.23 and 5.24, the head is in a good position and there has been satisfactory development in the acetabular roof

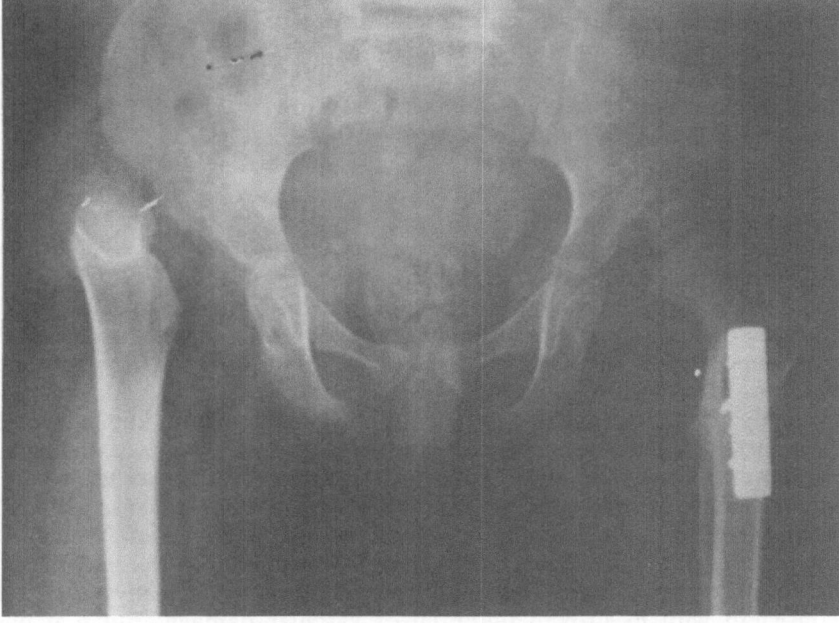

Fig. 5.26. Bilateral dislocations at the time of admission following multiple attempts at reduction as described

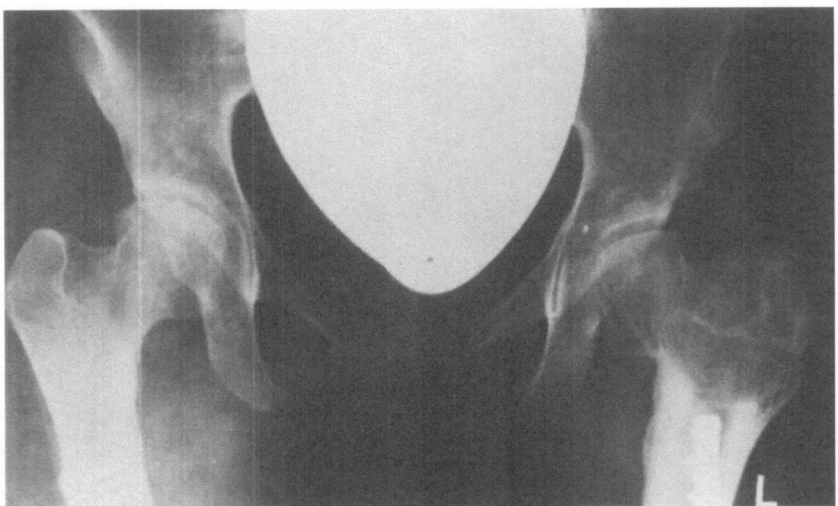

Fig. 5.27. Following the achievement of concentric reduction of both hips shown in Fig. 5.26 at open operation, both acetabula have developed as well as could be reasonably expected

Such evidence strongly suggests that given a chance the acetabulum will develop normally as long as irreversible damage has not been done to its growth potential (this may take much longer to occur than is generally supposed) and that there is no mechanical factor actively preventing it from doing so. The converse is also true. When it is seen that the acetabulum is not developing correctly it will not be because of a defect in the acetabulum but because of a mechanical failure of the joint as a whole. A unilateral dislocation was treated, in a girl aged 2 years, along routine lines. At the age of 7 it became apparent not only that no improvement had been achieved, but that there was some deterioration (Fig. 5.28). The radiograph showed that coxa valga had developed and that there was overgrowth of the lateral side of the head of the femur. Clinical examination showed that there had been a recurrence of the excessive angle of anteversion. Correction of these deformities allowed the hip to resume normal development, and to continue to grow normally, as seen at the age of 26 years (Fig. 5.29).

What would have happened if corrective osteotomy had not been carried out in time is open to conjecture. Unfortunately, similar hips (Fig. 5.30) have been encountered where an operation had not been carried out or had been delayed too long, with the inevitable deterioration of the joint beyond the point of no return (Fig. 5.31).

The mechanism involved in these changes is important. Why is it that some hips will develop normally while others deteriorate?

In any hip there is one of two types of movement. In both, the head of the femur is the centre of movement. In one the centre of the head is the centre around which all movements take place; this is concentric movement. In the other, while the head is still the centre of movement the centre of the head is not, because the head is slipping to and fro within the acetabulum. This is eccentric movement, which is the type of movement that constitutes subluxation. When concentric movement has been achieved the hip joint will be stable and will develop normally, or as normally as is consistent with its growth potential or vascular damage. But if it has not been achieved, and eccentric movement either persists or has developed, the hip will deteriorate, as shown by the progressive deterioration of the acetabulum seen

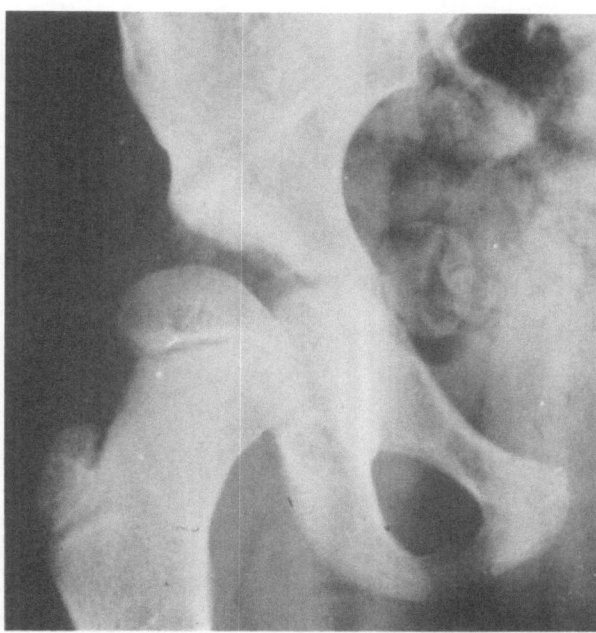

Fig. 5.28. Hip of a girl aged 7 years. The hip was originally treated at the age of 2 and for a while improved, but there has recently been progressive deterioration. Anteversion is present clinically and there is obvious coxa valga. The lateral part of the head has overgrown and the acetabulum is defective

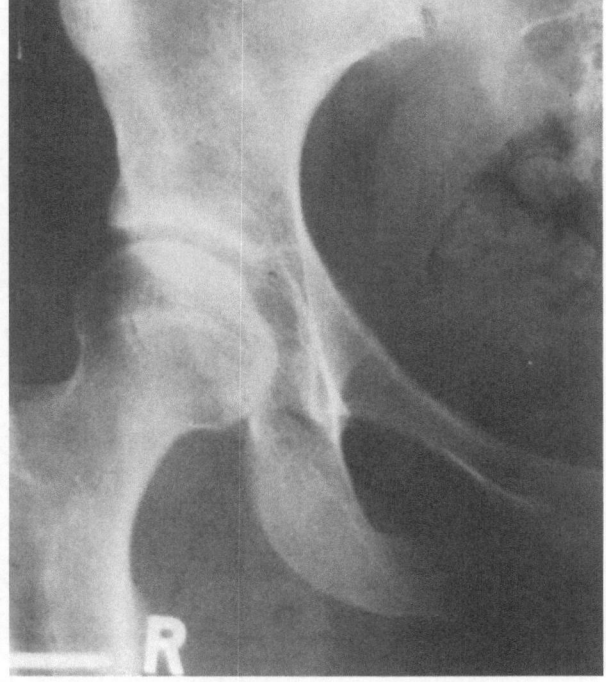

Fig. 5.29. The same hip as shown in Fig. 5.28 at the age of 26 following corrective osteotomy

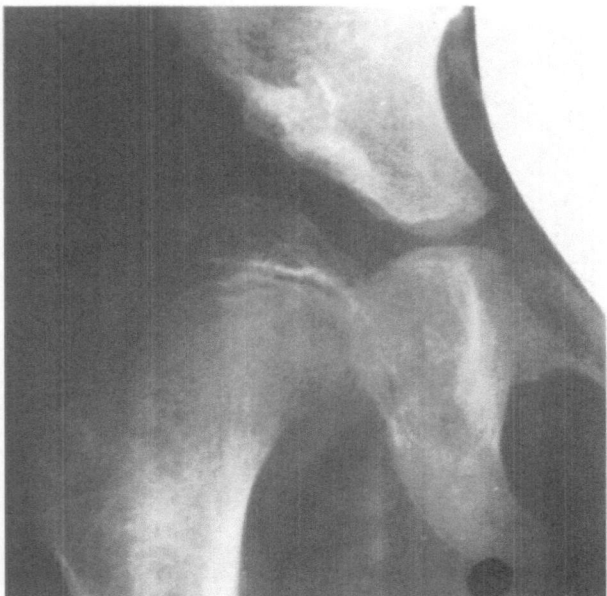

Fig. 5.30. A hip very similar to that seen in Fig. 5.28. No attempt was made to correct the mechanics

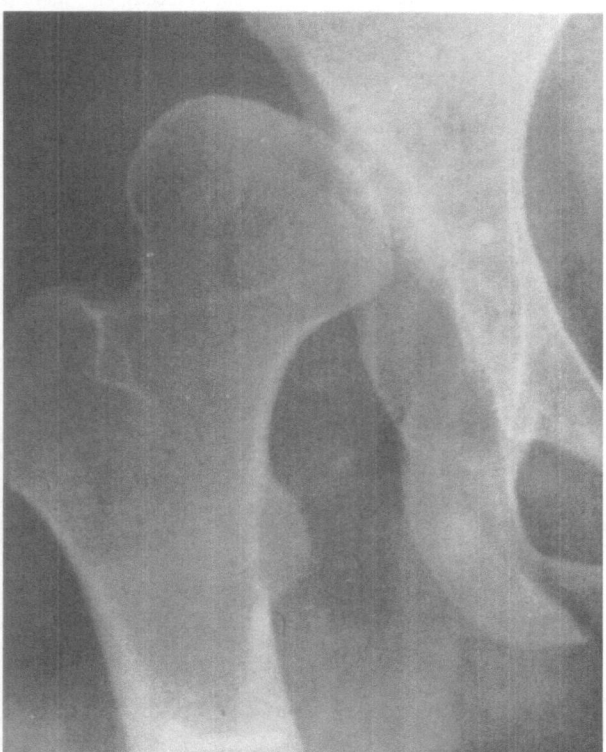

Fig. 5.31. Ten years later the damage to the hip shown in Fig. 5.30 is irreversible

radiologically. This appearance has often led to the mistaken belief that failure of the hip joint to develop normally is due to a failure of the acetabulum.

There is no reason why eccentric movement should not take place in any direction, but subluxation takes place anteriorly or anterosuperiorly, so that it seems likely that eccentric movement takes place in the anteroposterior plane. The action of the psoas muscle is closely connected with this movement. The action of the psoas can vary according to the shape of the upper end of the femur (Fig. 5.32). In the normal hip with a normal neck-shaft angle the axis of rotation is shown passing through the centre of the femoral head, through the centre of the knee joint, and down the tibia to the ground. This is the normal arrangement, and it is seen that the insertion of the psoas into the lower part of the lesser trochanter lies lateral to this axis, so that the psoas must be a medial rotator even though it is inserted into the femur posteromedially. In the second drawing (Fig. 5.32) the neck of the femur is valgus, or

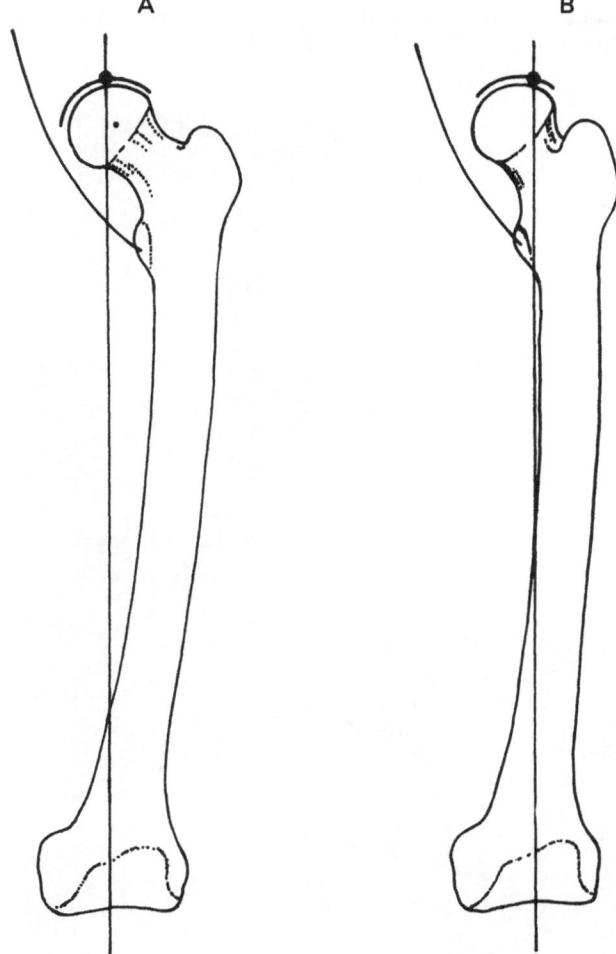

Fig. 5.32. Drawing illustrating the normal function of the psoas as a medial rotator (**A**), compared with the situation (**B**) in which anteversion and/or valgus have converted it into a lateral rotator

anteverted, or both, and it is clear that the insertion of the psoas is now medial to the axis of rotation so that the action of the psoas must be that of a lateral rotator. When the psoas is acting as a lateral rotator, every time it contracts to flex the hip it must try to rotate the femur laterally and will pull the femoral head against the anterior capsule. If the capsule is not lax and does not stretch no harm is done, but if it should become stretched, even by only a little at first, eccentric movement will be estab-lished and the hip will begin to deteriorate.

O'Malley (1963) recognised that the failure of the hip was due to the action of the psoas, and recommended simple division of the tendon. He was able to demonstrate considerable improvement after this procedure, because the deforming factor had been removed. But rather than divide the psoas it seems better to restore it to its original function as a medial rotator by carrying out the appropriate high femoral osteotomy and placing the neck markedly in a varus position. Then each time the psoas initiates flexion it will turn the head of the femur back into the acetabulum, removing any strain from the capsule. Slack will be taken up and concentric move-ment will be restored. The effect of this mechanism and its correction is well illustrated in Figs. 5.33 and 5.34.

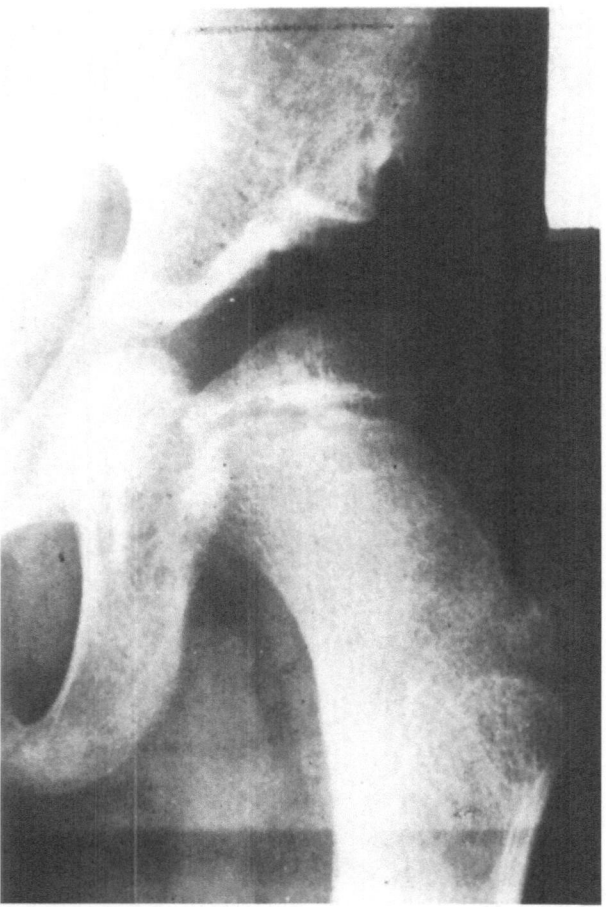

Fig. 5.33. The hip of a child aged 5 years, 2½ years after treatment. The hip is deteriorating

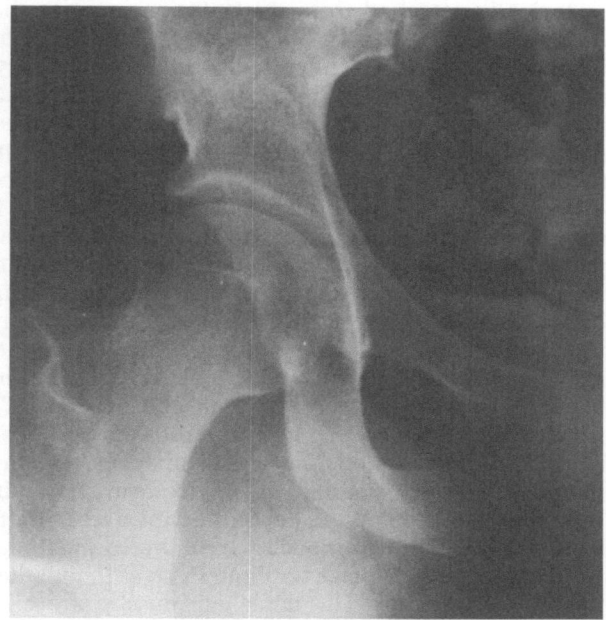

Fig. 5.34. The hip shown in Fig. 5.33 is normal 13 years after corrective osteotomy

A pelvic osteotomy correctly carried out will act in a similar way. The acetabulum will be tilted forwards over the front of the femoral head and will prevent forward displacement of the head. The operation will be rendered more effective by a capsuloplasty carried out at the same time (Chap. 6).

Causes of Mechanical Failure

Mechanical failure can occur as a result of abnormalities of soft tissues or of abnormalities of growth.

ABNORMALITIES OF SOFT TISSUES

Capsular Contracture

Very occasionally a hip is encountered in which the initial reduction on the frame or by other means is exceptionally difficult. Subsequent open operation and excision of the limbus is also exceptionally difficult. The postoperative radiograph shows that the head of the femur is standing out, which is not uncommon in the first postoperative radiograph, owing to postoperative swelling, and is not significant. But the head is also slightly high, which is pathological. Removal of the plaster and attempts at manipulative reduction are useless, and should not be attempted. As soon as the postoperative reaction is over the hip must be re-explored.

Operation   The small incision used for excision of the limbus must be extended across the front of the groin, almost to the tendon of the adductor longus. The sartorius is detached from the anterior superior iliac spine with a small piece of cartilage, which will make re-attachment easier. The femoral nerve is dissected out, as is the femoral artery. The nerve is retracted laterally and the vessels medially. The rectus muscle is detached with a small piece of cartilage and is turned down. If still more room is required the ileopsoas muscle can be mobilised by detaching the iliacus from the iliac crest. The whole of the front of the joint, with the transverse incision in the capsule from the previous operation, will be exposed. The head of the femur is dislocated from the acetabulum so that the whole of the acetabulum is visible. If it is apparent that the technique of the previous operation was at fault and that the medial part of the capsule was inadequately divided or that the transverse ligament'is still intact it can be corrected without difficulty; but it is unlikely that this will be found to be the cause of the trouble. A finger introduced across the joint will probably feel tight contracted bands in the posterior capsule and it will not be possible until these have been divided for the head to be fully reduced. This is a procedure which is bound to cause some anxiety because it must be done 'blind', by touch, and the sciatic nerve will be close to the cutting scissors. But as the incision is made almost in line with the nerve and there will be no previous scarring, the danger is probably more apparent than real. The virtue of this anterior exposure is that it enables the surgeon to see that the reduction is complete beyond doubt, rather than having to assume that it is, as when a more lateral approach is used. In closing the wound the capsule is closed with stout catgut sutures placed obliquely, so as to pull the distal cut edge medially and so tighten the capsule. The detached muscles are all re-attached and the wound is closed. Subsequent treatment is continued as though the problem had never been encountered, but after such an extensive dissection mobilisation is bound to be slow. This slowness of mobilisation may sometimes be helped by converting the plaster spica into broomstick plasters for 2 weeks before the osteotomy is performed (Fig. 5.35).

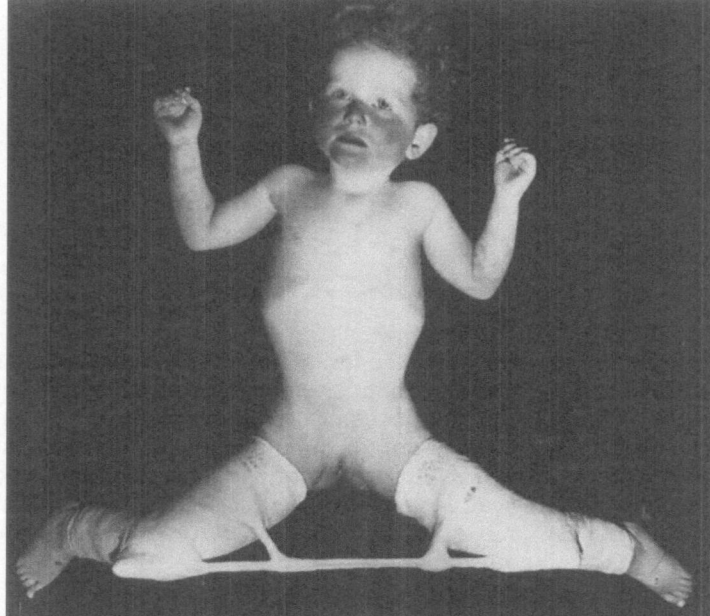

Fig. 5.35. Child in broomstick plasters

Intracapsular Adhesions

Intracapsular adhesions are a common complication in the hip which has previously been treated; usually with open operation, but where reduction has not been achieved (Fig. 5.36). In these circumstances adhesions will develop between the neck of the femur and the capsule (Putti, cited in Hass 1948). These adhesions may even extend onto the articular surface of the head. When this happens the effective capsule is greatly shortened, so that there is only a limited range of movement and this will not be sufficient to permit reduction (Fig. 5.37). It is these adhesions which

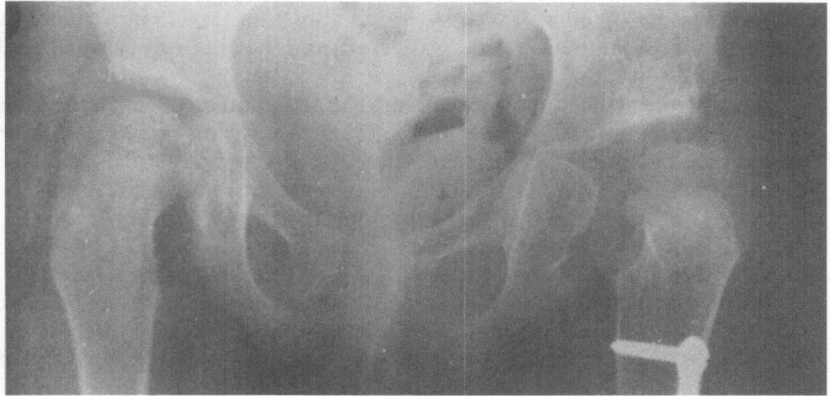

Fig. 5.36. Following multiple attempts at reduction this hip is held in a position of displacement with full lateral rotation by intra-articular adhesions

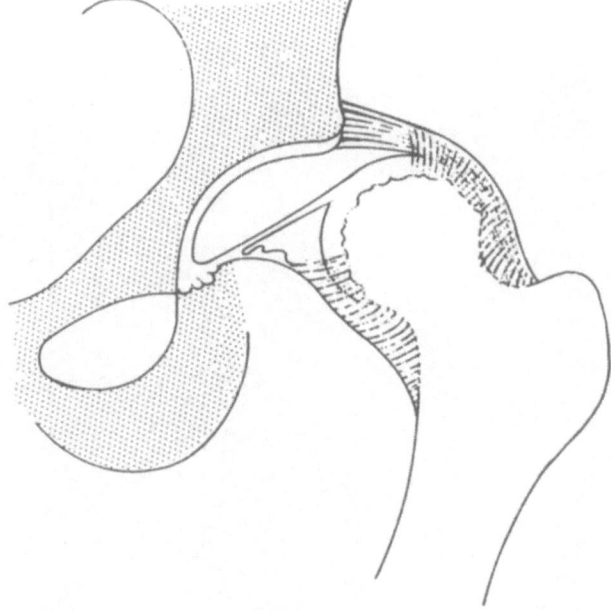

Fig. 5.37. Drawing showing how intra-articular adhesions prevent reduction in hips such as that shown in Fig. 5.36

are effectively holding the head out of the acetabulum. Separating them from the neck will endanger the blood supply to the ossific nucleus. The most satisfactory form of treatment is the circumferential division of the capsule, carried out through the anterior approach already described. The operation should be postponed for a short while until the child has tried to gain some mobility. The capsule is then freed as far as possible from surrounding scar tissue and is divided circumferentially as close as possible to the lip of the acetabulum. The head of the femur is dislocated from the acetabulum and any scar tissue in the acetabulum is removed. It is interesting that while the adhesions frequently involve the head of the femur and produce quite extensive pitting and damage to the articular cartilage, in the acetabulum the cartilage is seldom involved, nor is there appreciable damage to it. Usually the damage to the acetabulum is much less than expected, and the shape of the acetabulum is within reasonable limits.

After this wide division of the capsule the head can be reduced into the acetabulum without using force (Figs. 5.38 and 5.39) in a position of full medial rotation. The capsule will then come to lie in a new position so that when the incision heals it will be holding the head of the femur in the joint instead of holding it out as was previously the case. It is wise to put a stout double stitch through the lip of the acetabulum anteriorly and through the capsule to ensure a good position. The hip is immobilised in medial rotation and abduction with a hip spica for 1 month. If as a result of the persistent displacement anteversion has recurred it will need to be corrected by osteotomy, but this is by no means always the case. Should it be necessary it will be wise to allow 2 weeks in broomstick plasters to encourage mobilisation before embarking on the second operation. After these operations mobilisation is bound to be slow, and although it can be expected that at least 90° of flexion will be achieved it is unlikely that there will be a full range.

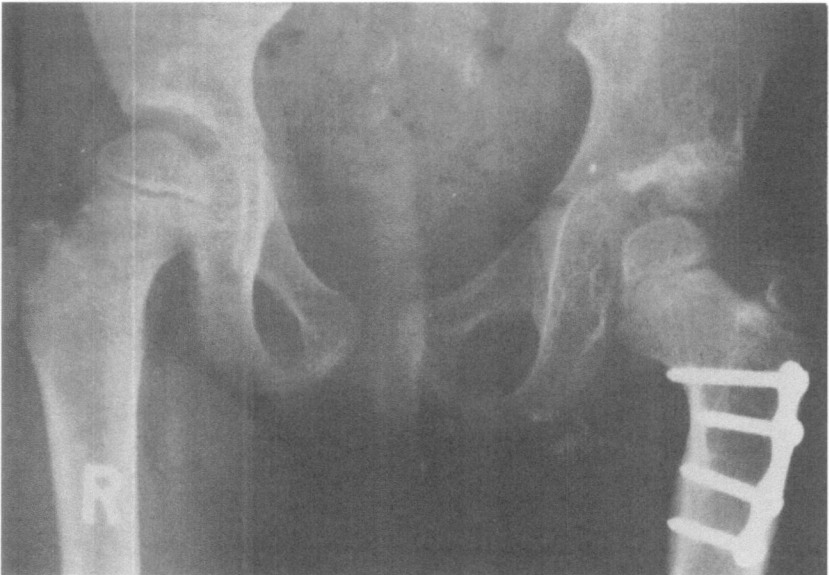

Fig. 5.38. Concentric reduction of the hip shown in Fig. 5.36 was achieved by open reduction with circumferential division of the capsule and has been maintained, as seen 2 years later

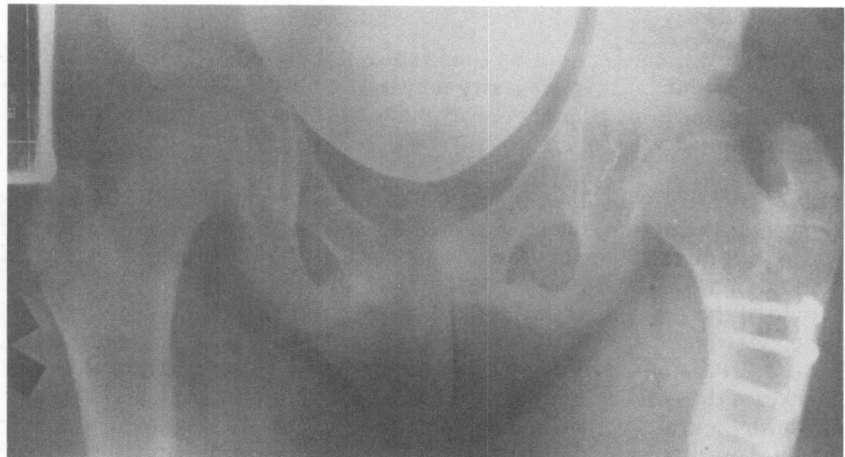

Fig. 5.39. Four years after the state illustrated in Fig. 5.38, the hip is continuing to develop well

Extra-articular Contractures

Adductor Muscles   Very occasionally during mobilisation a contracture may develop in the adductor muscles; if this is sufficient to maintain the hip in some adduction or even to prevent the hip from abducting beyond the neutral, the mother should be instructed in how to stretch the tight muscle manually without using such force as to cause damage. Usually this is all that is required, because the contracture is no more than a temporary spasm which will pass. If, however, the deformity persists and appears to be doing damage to the hip a tenotomy must be performed and the leg held in wide abduction in a plaster spica for 2 weeks, followed by a resumption of normal activities. Night splintage has not been necessary but would do no harm if the abduction was not too extreme.

Abductor Muscles   While an adductor contracture does damage to the same hip an abductor contracture does damage to the opposite hip. This needs watching most carefully during the mobilisation of bilaterally dislocated hips. No hip in a small child will tolerate adduction, even though of minor degree, for long without showing signs of deterioration, even if the hip was initially normal. Damage will be even more marked if the hip has been previously dislocated.

During mobilisation of bilateral dislocations a close watch must be kept to be sure that both hips are adducting at the same rate. If it becomes apparent that one hip is regaining adduction more rapidly than the other, and if this is not corrected, damage even to the point of dislocation may be done to it because it will adduct to lie beside the other, which is abducted. If it is seen that one hip is mobilising more rapidly than the other, the more mobile hip should be immobilised in some abduction in a single hip spica until the other has caught up. It was noticed when the bilaterally dislocated hips were reviewed that in one this mechanism had led to complete dislocation, and that in those where one hip had developed slightly less well than the other there had often been persistence of a minor degree of abduction on the good side, sometimes so slight that it would pass unnoticed unless specifically looked for. This mechanism will be considered again when leg length inequality is discussed.

Capsular Laxity

Because soft tissues cannot be seen radiologically it is all too easy to underestimate their importance. Capsular laxity may easily be overlooked as a cause of displacement when the bony changes are so much more obvious. The laxity may be transitory or persistent.

Transitory   It is not uncommon for there to be some laxity for a while after the completion of treatment (Fig. 5.40). Such an appearance may cause unnecessary alarm; it is due to some degree of capsular laxity still persisting from the dislocation, combined with the loss of muscle tone inevitable after a period of treatment. Provided the mechanics of the joint have been properly corrected there is no cause for concern and the hip will develop normally (Fig. 5.41). In such a condition any form of treatment involving rest in recumbency, or worse still splintage, will either aggravate the condition or perpetuate it by making the muscles even more toneless, and with the child lying in bed the leg will be in lateral rotation and the deformity may increase until real pathology has developed. The child should be encouraged to mobilise and to start weight-bearing as soon as possible. The child will do this better at home than in hospital, and the temptation to take unnecessary radiographs will be reduced. The child should not be given a further appointment for 3 months, or better still 6.

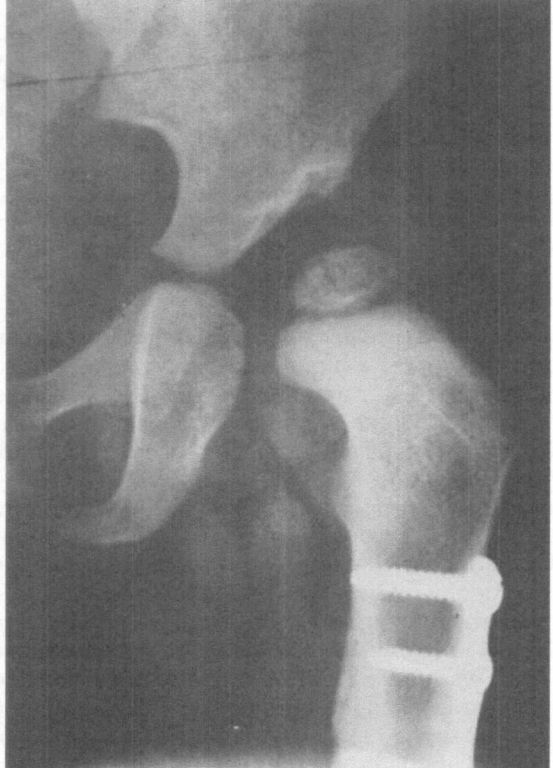

Fig. 5.40. Three months after removal of the final plaster the capsule of this hip is lax, permitting some minor degree of displacement

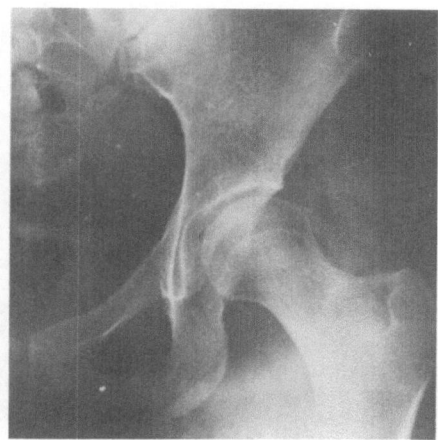

Fig. 5.41. The same hip as shown in Fig. 5.40, seen 18 years later. No treatment was carried out and the hip is now normal

Persistent   Persistent laxity is a much more serious problem. Very occasionally it may be seen after perfectly straightforward treatment, but it is most commonly seen after complications have occurred involving multiple operations on the joint which have resulted in much scarring and fibrosis of the capsule so that spontaneous shrinkage cannot occur.

A child was found to have a dislocated hip at the age of 20 months. Attempts at closed reduction failed, and open reduction was undertaken on three occasions, followed each time by a period in plaster. A high femoral osteotomy failed to stabilise the hip, which remained displaced (Fig. 5.42). The child was admitted to The Nuffield Orthopaedic Centre at the age of 3 years. She was found to walk with a very severe limp and to walk and lie with the leg in full lateral rotation. There was an excellent range of movement in all directions, and when the leg was gently rotated medially into neutral rotation a radiograph showed that the displacement was completely reduced without any effort (Fig. 5.43). The radiograph showed that there had already been severe damage to the blood supply to the ossific nucleus and to a lesser extent to the growth plate; deformity was therefore inevitable, but it would be much worse if the displacement was allowed to persist.

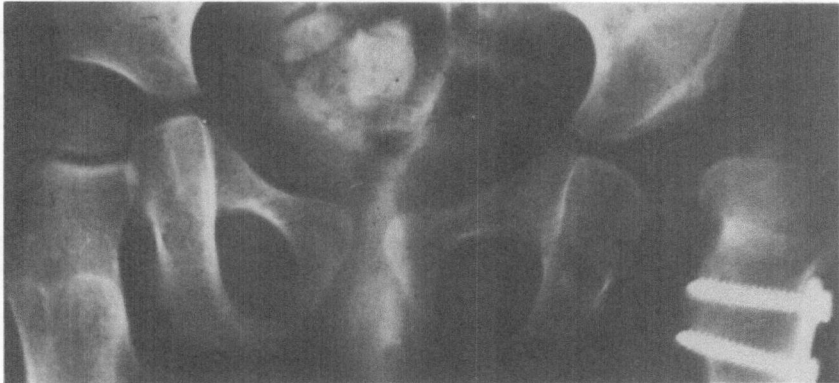

Fig. 5.42. The displacement in this hip is due to persistent capsular laxity, the result of multiple open reductions

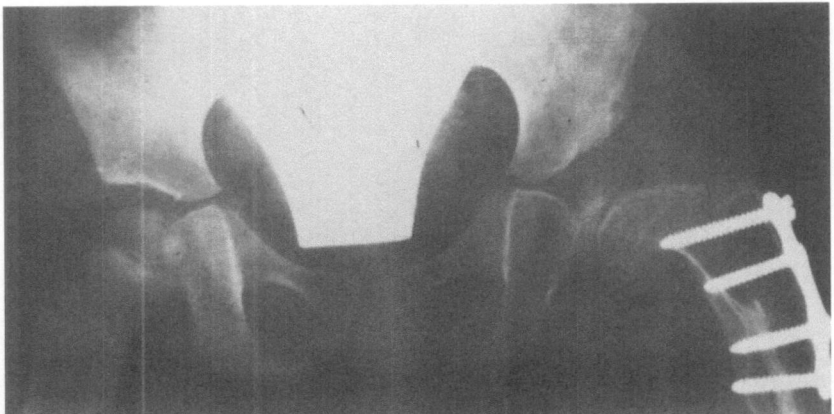

Fig. 5.43. The hip shown in Fig. 5.42 was reduced very easily by medial rotation

Through the anterior approach already described the anterior part of the capsule was exposed, an ellipse was excised close to the lip of the acetabulum, and the free margin of the capsule was sutured with stout catgut stitches to the lip of the acetabulum, through which the stitches were passed. The sutures were tied with the hip held in full medial rotation. Although the inevitable deformity of the head and neck developed complete reduction was established (Fig. 5.44) and has lasted for 20 years.

Abnormalities of Growth

Abnormalities of growth may result either from damage to the growth plate or from interference with the circulation. They may lead to valgus, varus, increased anteversion, shortening of the femoral neck, or overgrowth of the whole leg with leg length inequality.

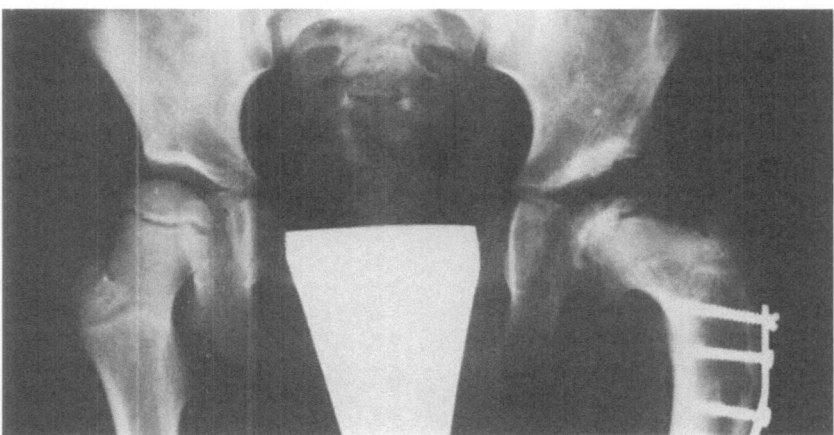

Fig. 5.44. Three years after simple capsular plication the hip shown in Figs. 5.42 and 5.43 has remained reduced

Valgus and Anteversion   The most common growth deformity is coxa valga. The likely causes of this are over-stimulation of the capital end of the metaphysis due to unfamiliar pressure following reduction; under-stimulation of the outer end of the metaphysis resulting from weakness of the abductor muscles; and a combination of the two. The deformity may be associated with enlargement of the lateral part of the capital epiphysis, for the reasons already described. It is a deformity of overgrowth and for this reason is not associated with ischaemia, which would lead to coxa vara.

If the possible development of valgus is anticipated and the neck of the femur is put into more than 10°–15° varus to avoid this, often exactly the opposite effect from that hoped for will result and valgus will develop even more quickly. As has already been noted the development may lead to an eccentric type of movement, causing deterioration in the acetabulum and progressive displacement; but this is not necessarily the case and normal development of the acetabulum is quite consistent with an excessive degree of valgus (Fig. 5.45) provided that eccentric movement does not occur. Not infrequently when the hip has developed normally in spite of coxa valga it will be found that towards the end of growth the neck-shaft angle improves (Fig. 5.46).

The reason for the recurrence of anteversion is by no means clear, but it does recur in about 20% of hips and is often associated with valgus; it is very uncommon for anteversion to develop in the presence of varus. Anteversion will develop as the result of eccentric movement, which may have resulted from the coxa valga or from persistent joint laxity; but this is not the only cause; recurrent anteversion may be found in a hip which is growing normally, and the development of anteversion may on occasion be the initiating factor in the production of eccentric movement. Also anteversion has continued to recur in spite of as many as three corrections until the end of growth. It seems therefore that there is in some hips a built-in mechanism for the development of anteversion.

A possible explanation is that either as part of the original deformity or as a result of treatment the metaphysis becomes twisted so that the capital end of it is not only facing upwards but is also facing forwards to some extent (Fig. 5.47).

Although such a mechanism is difficult to prove, there are two things in favour of this explanation. Firstly, if the metaphysis is directed upwards and forwards the two

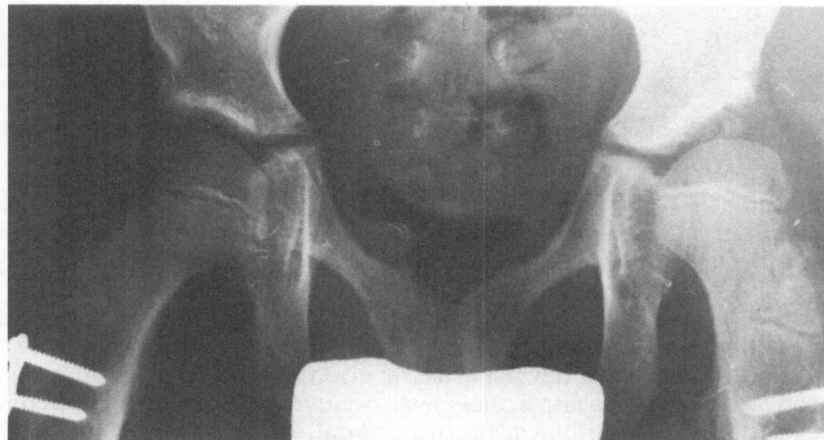

Fig. 5.45. Following treatment, marked valgus has developed in these bilateral dislocations, but the heads are well placed and the acetabula are developing. There is no indication for further treatment

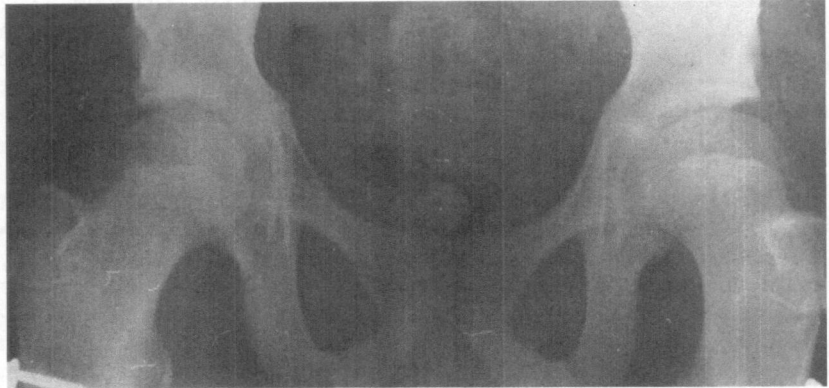

Fig. 5.46. Six years later the right hip is normal and the left is almost so in spite of the coxa valga

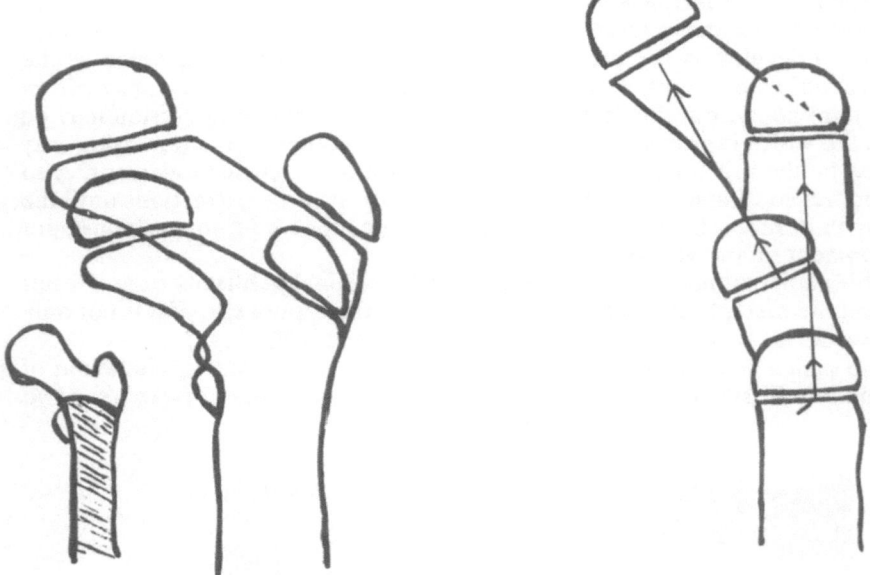

Fig. 5.47. Illustration of a suggested mechanism for the recurrence of anteversion combined with valgus

deformities would be expected to develop at the same time, which is often found to be the case; and secondly, if anteversion has developed once it is not uncommon for it to do so again after correction, even though on the second occasion it may not reach the point where treatment is required because the end of growth may have been reached. This suggests that the mechanism causing anteversion has persisted and in fact continues as long as growth in some cases.

Again, the fact that anteversion has recurred and has persisted does not necessarily mean that progressive displacement will occur, even though it may be combined with valgus; but such a hip must be suspect and will need watching. If deterioration appears treatment must be undertaken because there would inevitably be further deterioration otherwise (Figs. 5.28 and 5.29).

An unusual type of coxa valga has been seen several times. The appearance suggests that there has been some interference with growth of the upper border of the neck, causing the head to tilt into valgus. This deformity, which has only been seen on a few occasions, has not become apparent before the age of 10 years, which makes it difficult to understand when the damage could have been done. Figure 5.48 shows the hip of a child aged 11 years, in whom the acetabulum is developing well; there is a little bulging of the lateral part of the femoral head; the upper border of the femoral neck is slightly irregular but it is a good length. But 3 years later, at the age of 14 (Fig. 5.49), the femoral head has tilted into valgus so that the distance between the head and the greater trochanter is greatly reduced. This has had no effect on the development of the hip, which is almost normal. This is not always the case, as can be seen in Fig. 5.50, where subluxation had developed with a similar deformity and had to be corrected by a varus osteotomy (Fig. 5.51).

Because treatment consists of correction of the deformity it is important to determine in advance what it is. Is it valgus only? Is it anteversion only? Or is it a combination of the two? The differentiation between the deformities can be made more readily by clinical examination than is possible by radiography. With radiography it is difficult to determine degrees of rotation when the neck is in valgus, and the more marked the valgus position the more difficult it becomes. Clinically the arc of rotation of the extended hip can be taken as a reasonably good guide to the angle of anteversion in a child. With no anteversion the arc is roughly 45° of both medial and lateral rotation. As the angle of anteversion increases so does the arc of medial rotation, while lateral rotation decreases. With 45° of anteversion medial rotation will be 90° and lateral rotation will be nil. The neck-shaft angle can be ascertained from a plain anteroposterior radiograph taken with the hip in full medial rotation.

From these simple investigations it will be possible to decide what form the osteotomy will take. The technique for rotation and varus osteoomy has already been described and is basically the same for the larger child or adolescent as for the small child.

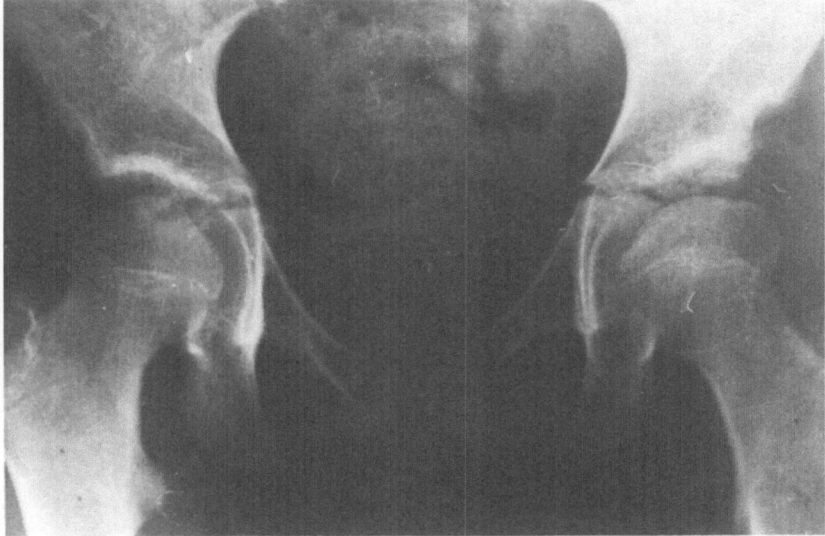

Fig. 5.48. The hip of a child aged 12, ten years after treatment

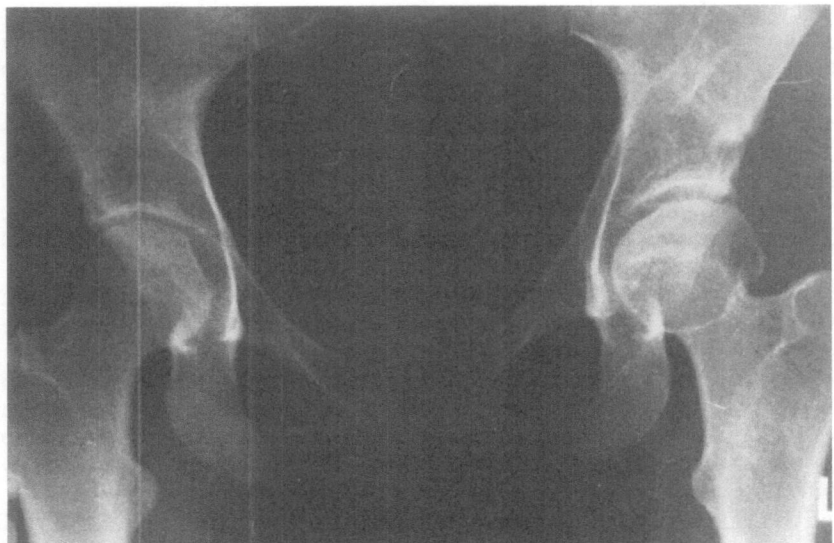

Fig. 5.49. Three years later the appearance of the hip shown in Fig. 5.48 suggests interference with growth on the lateral aspect of the neck causing tilting of the capital epiphysis. The acetabulum has developed normally

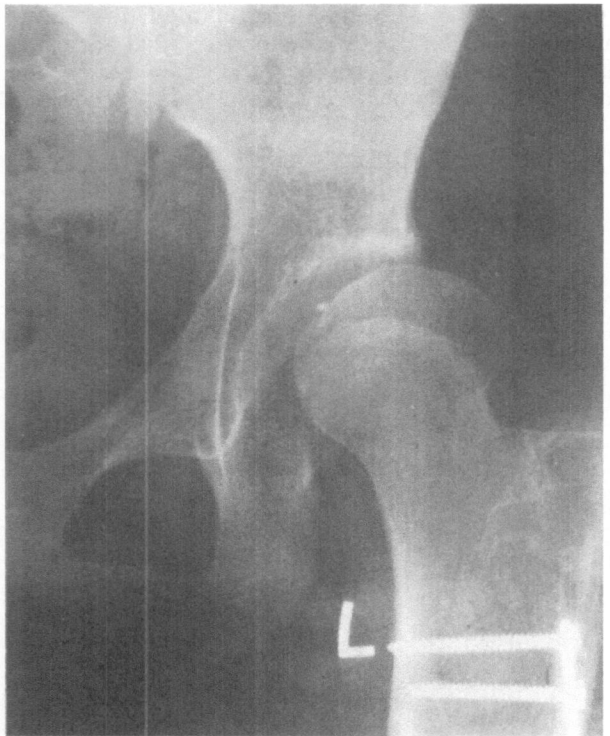

Fig. 5.50. A similar condition to that seen in Figs. 5.48 and 5.49, which has developed with subluxation. Which came first is uncertain

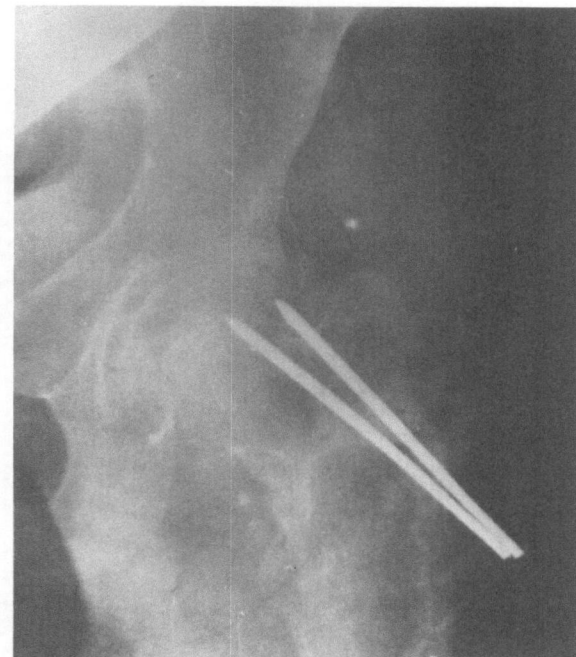

Fig. 5.51. The same hip as shown in Fig. 5.50, after a varus osteotomy performed with an iliac wedge. The subluxation was reduced but in later years gradually recurred as the deformity increased

Varus Osteotomy (Fig. 5.52)

The type of osteotomy best suited to a particular case will depend on the leg length. The production of varus will make the leg shorter, and the removal of a medial wedge will make it shorter still. Often this is desirable because in many hips in which late subluxation is developing there has been quite a marked overgrowth, and this overgrowth may in itself have contributed to the subluxation by putting the hip into some adduction when the child is standing. An operation which shortens the leg is often advantageous. On a few occasions the lengthening has been of such a degree that a combination of varus and an inner wedge has not been sufficient to produce equalisation and it has been necessary to remove a trapezoid.

The osteotomy should be made as high as possible, the natural flare of the greater trochanter being exploited so that the apparent deformity will be reduced to a minimum. Through a lateral incision the lateral aspect of the upper end of the femur is exposed up to the prominence of the greater trochanter. If a plate is still present from the previous treatment it should be removed. If the configuration of the upper end of the femur is such that it is possible to remove a medial wedge above the lesser trochanter and to apply a small plate with the two upper screws above the oesteotomy, then the plate is best placed on the lateral aspect of the femur. A Steinmann's pin is inserted immediately below the prominence and directed horizontally. A plate is slotted onto the pin through the upper hole, and the plate is laid along the femur. A second pin is inserted horizontally parallel to the first, and through the upper hole in the lower part of the plate. The plate is removed. The bone is divided transversely as high as possible, allowing just enough room for the two screws above.

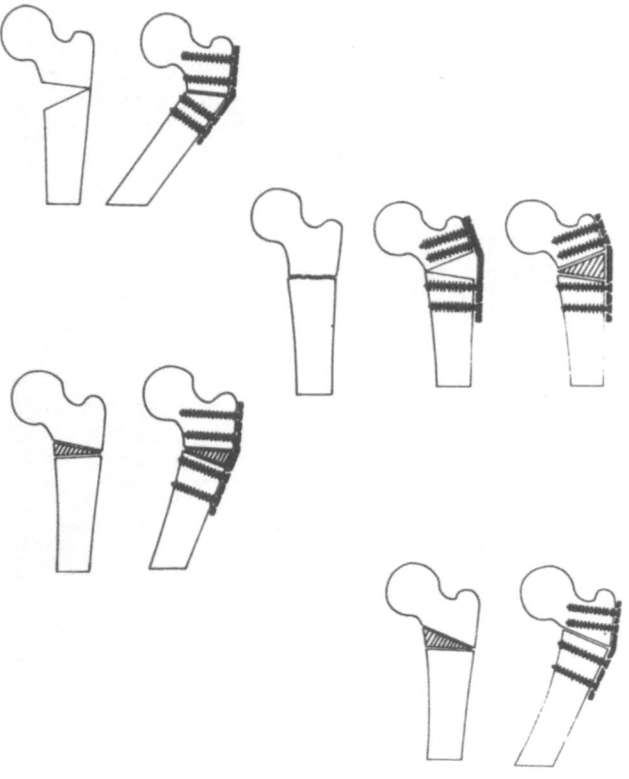

Fig. 5.52. Drawings to demonstrate the different types of varus osteotomies which can be used so as to influence leg length

When the transverse division is half-way through the bone the second cut is started at an angle to the first equal to the required increase in varus. Care must be taken to ensure that the cuts are in the same plane, so that the wedge will not be either anteromedial or posteromedial. The upper cut, which is started first, should be completed first. If the lower cut is completed first there will be no means of controlling the upper fragment while the upper cut is completed. The wedge can then be removed in one piece and the two fragments, controlled by the pins, can be brought together. The plate is then angled to fit the lateral aspect of the femur and is slotted onto the pins and screwed in position as has been previously described. The plate does not need to be large; it is there only to ensure maintenance of the position and not to provide rigid fixation, and for this reason a plaster spica must be applied. Attempts to rely on internal fixation alone have proved difficult, and it is only in these cases that complications have arisen. At the age of 7 union will be sound in 6 weeks; at 10 union will take 8 weeks; and at 12 it will take up to 12 weeks.

If the varus osteotomy with removal of medial wedge seems likely to shorten the femur too much a wedge of half the estimated size is removed medially, reversed, and put in the outer side (Fig. 5.53). If the shortening will still be too much the whole correction may be obtained by making a single transverse osteotomy which is opened up on the outer side, an angled plate being applied without any bone being inserted. Up to the age of 13 or 14 this will not interfere with union, but over this age it is probably wise to introduce a graft taken from the pelvis (Fig. 5.51).

If it is not possible to apply the plate sufficiently high on the lateral aspect of the femur it may be applied anteriorly. The anterior aspect of the upper end of the femur is exposed, the clearance extending onto the neck of the femur. Pins are inserted to make control of the fragments easier, and the bone is divided between them as high as is possible, allowing room for two screws above the osteotomy: the required angulation is obtained and the plate is applied (Figs. 5.54–5.56).

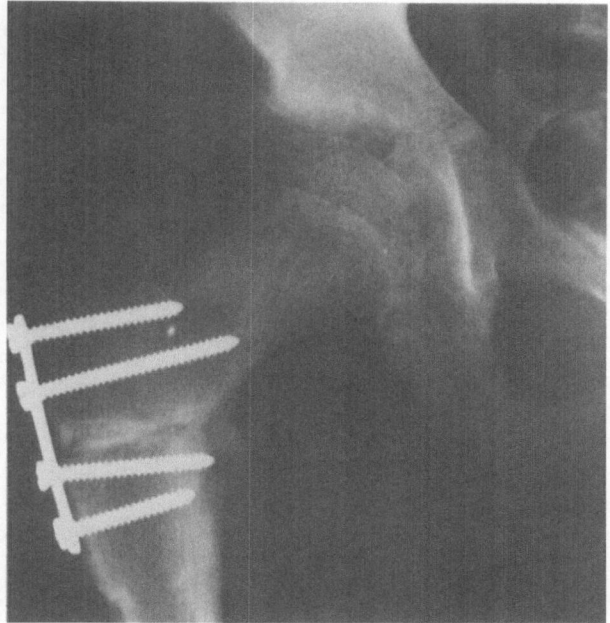

Fig. 5.53. Varus has been obtained at an osteotomy by removing a medial wedge and inserting it laterally

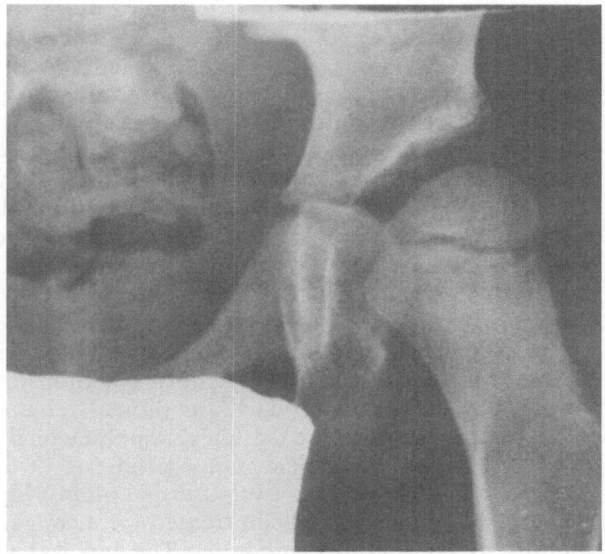

Fig. 5.54. Severe valgus in this joint is affecting the development of the acetabulum

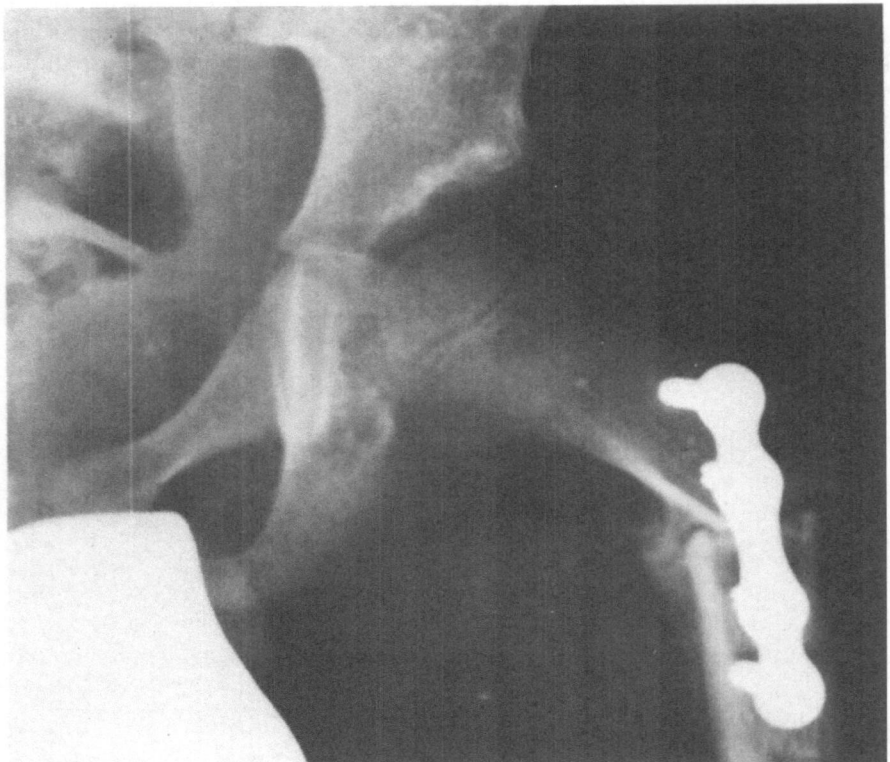

Fig. 5.55. A varus osteotomy has been carried out as high as possible for correction of the joint shown in Fig. 5.54, and the plate is applied anteriorly

Osteotomy Combining Rotation and Varus   Rotation can be combined with varus in the same oesteotomy in two ways. The simplest is to proceed as in the small child, introducing the two pins at the angle required to provide the estimated degree of rotation. When the wedge is removed, the major portion of material is taken from the lower fragment where the point of the lower pin emerges, which will become the medial side if the upper pin has been placed accurately in the lateral aspect of the femur. The difficulty is that in the older child the cortex will be too hard for the wedge to be removed with bone nibblers and it will have to be removed with a saw. The alternative is to make the lower osteotomy transverse and to remove all of the wedge from the upper fragment (Fig. 5.52). When the wedge is closed it will be possible to rotate the lower fragment on the upper without altering the alignment. If a wedge is opened up instead of being closed this difficulty will not arise.

. One of the advantages of the femoral osteotomy is that the leg can be shortened by varying amounts as required without difficulty, but with the pelvic osteotomy there is a tendency to lengthen the leg. This is a point which must be taken into account when the type of operation is being considered.

Age need not be a bar to a femoral osteotomy. Figure 5.57 shows the hip of a child 13 years of age who had been treated for a congenital dislocation at the age of 18 months by conservative methods. The hip was subluxated, the acetabulum was defective, and the girl limped badly and had some pain. A varus osteotomy was performed (Fig. 5.58) and 21 years later there is full range of movement, no limp, and no pain. The radiograph shows that there has been no further displacement and there is little if any evidence of stress (Fig. 5.59). This indicates that in spite of the appearance the hip must be stable and there must be concentric movement.

Leg Inequality

As already stated, persistent adduction of the hip in a young child may have a deleterious effect on the way in which the adducted hip grows. Inequality of leg length will produce persistent adduction of the long leg and abduction of the short, with the result that the hip on the side of the short leg will benefit and the hip on the side of the long leg will be adversely affected. Sometimes the leg on the affected side will be short, for a while at least, but provided the shortening is no more than ¾ in. no raise need be put on the shoe because the shortening will do nothing but good; but if the affected leg grows too long, as is more usual, a raise must always be put on the other shoe. There have been cases in which the overgrowth has been such that it has

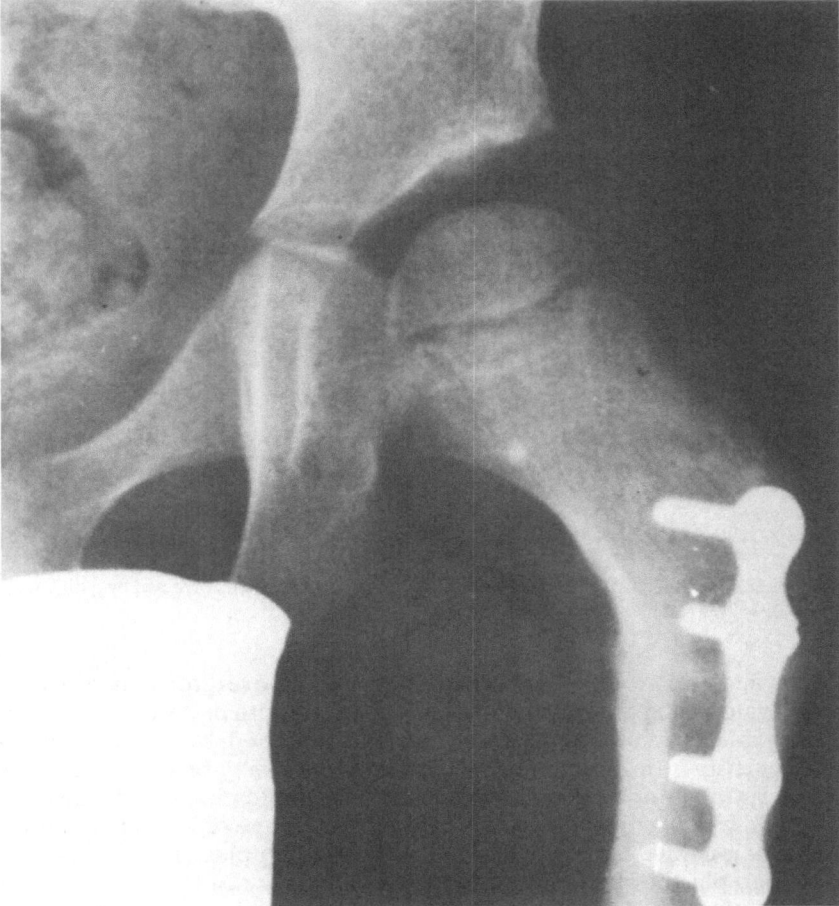

Fig. 5.56. The hip 2 years after the osteotomy shown in Fig. 5.55

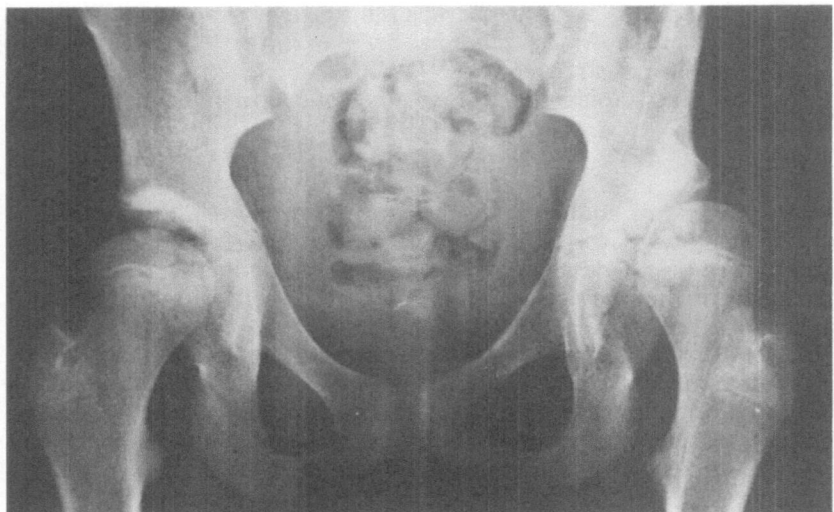

Fig. 5.57. Hips of a girl of 13. The left hip has been previously treated conservatively. The left femoral neck is valgus and there is subluxatioh with failure of acetabular development. The right hip is also a little dysplastic with a CE angle of 10° but the 'dew-drop' is normal

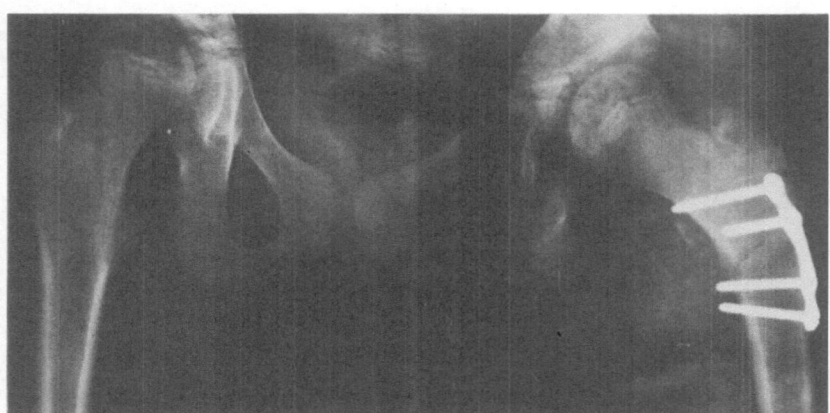

Fig. 5.58. The valgus and anteversion seen in Fig. 5.57 have been corrected by a high femoral osteotomy

been necessary to shorten the leg surgically. But overgrowth is very often associated with valgus, and the valgus and overgrowth can both be corrected at the same time by a suitable varus osteotomy or, as already mentioned, by the removal of a trapezoid.

Sometimes the shortening of the affected leg may be enough to actually damage the previously normal hip or at least give the impression that damage has been done. A child was found to have a dislocated hip at the age of 1 year and was treated for this by manipulative reduction and 8 months in a frog plaster. At the age of 2½ years the radiograph showed that there was still some displacement, with well-marked ischaemic chaiges in the ossific nucleus and possibly damage to the growth plate. A rotation osteotomy corrected the displacement (Fig. 5.60). Shortly afterwards the child was lost to follow-up and was not seen again until 12 years later, when she was referred back from another part of the country because of the appearance of the left hip, which had previously been normal (Fig. 5.61). This radiograph shows that the pelvis is tilted because the right femur has become shortened by 2½ in. as the result of damage to the growth plate at the initial treatment.

The appearance of the right hip has been greatly improved by levelling the pelvis with a 2½ in. raise under the right foot (Fig. 5.62). The acetabulum has certainly been damaged, but before contemplating surgical correction of the acetabulum leg equalisation should be undertaken to see whether the left hip will improve sufficiently when the deforming factor has been removed.

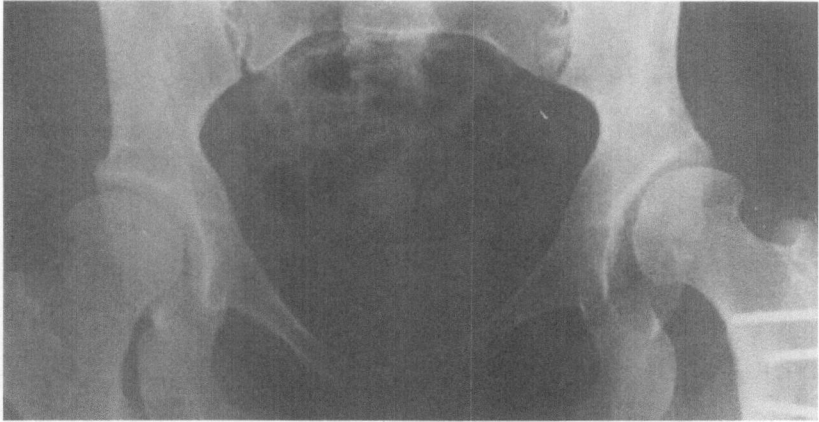

Fig. 5.59. Twenty years after high femoral osteotomy the left hip seen in Figs. 5.57 or 5.58 is showing no sign of displacement or wear and the right hip with the slight dysplasia is still showing no evidence of deterioration even though the CE angle is only 10°

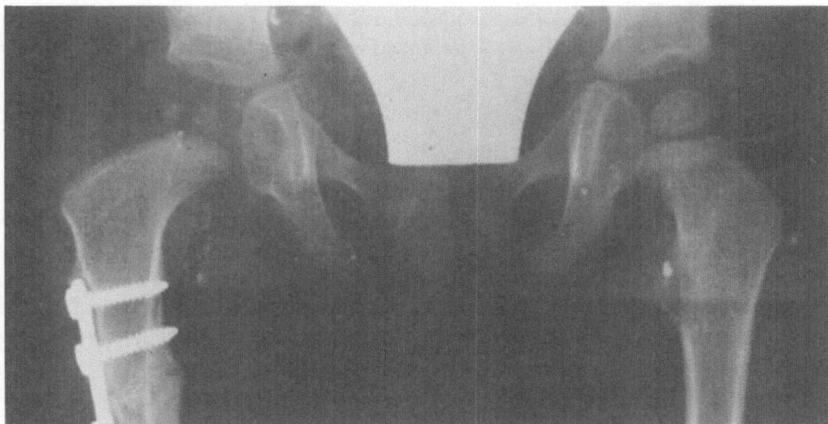

Fig. 5.60. Following initial manipulative treatment of this hip there is severe vascular and growth disturbance on the right

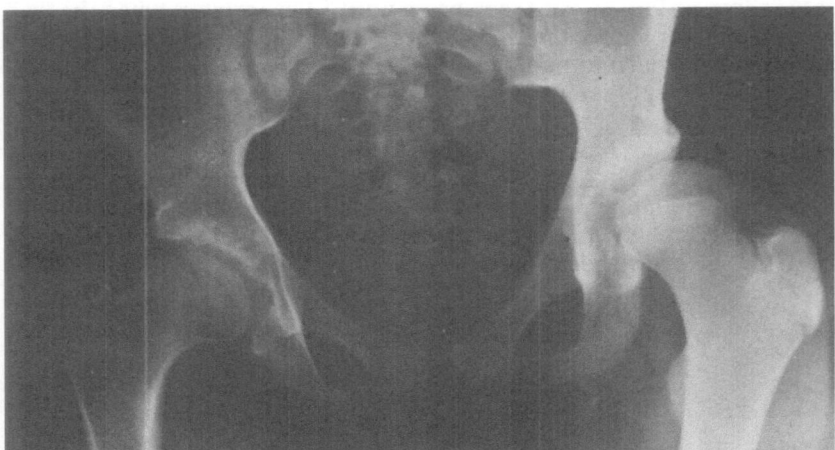

Fig. 5.61. Twelve years after the initial treatment of the hips shown in Fig. 5.60 there is marked tilting of the pelvis due to 2½ in. shortening of the right femur. The right hip has benefited from the shortening because it is abducted, but the left hip has been damaged by being adducted. The appearance on the left suggests subluxation

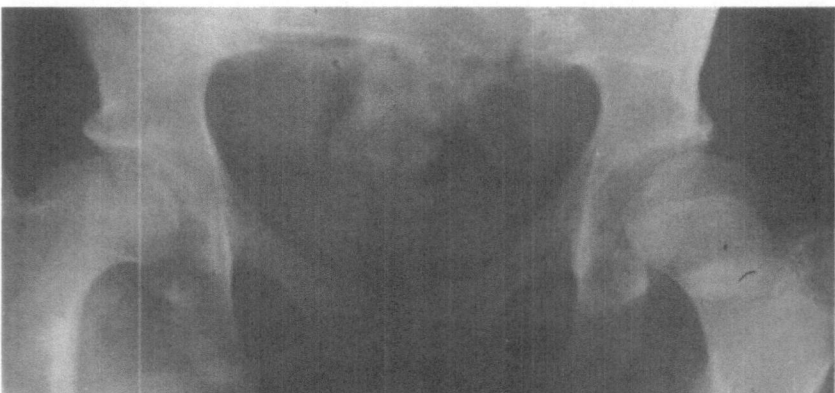

Fig. 5.62. The appearance of the left hip seen in Fig. 5.61 is much improved by levelling of the pelvis

Persistent Varus

A varus deformity will usually correct itself spontaneously in congenital dislocation of the hip but not in Perthes' disease. Sometimes it will become over-corrected so that valgus will develop. This is much less likely to happen as the child gets older, so that by the age of 10 care must be taken not to produce too marked a degree of varus at osteotomy, because it may persist. This is because in very early childhood the upper end of the femur, as can be seen from the Harris's lines, grows quickly but after the age of 5 the rate of growth slows considerably.

Occasionally coxa vara develops as a growth deformity (Fig. 5.63). In such cases there is a marked varus which develops to the extent shown but no further. But it does not correct. If it is thought that the deformity is too great it must be corrected by operation. This deformity, which is a growth disturbance, must not be confused with

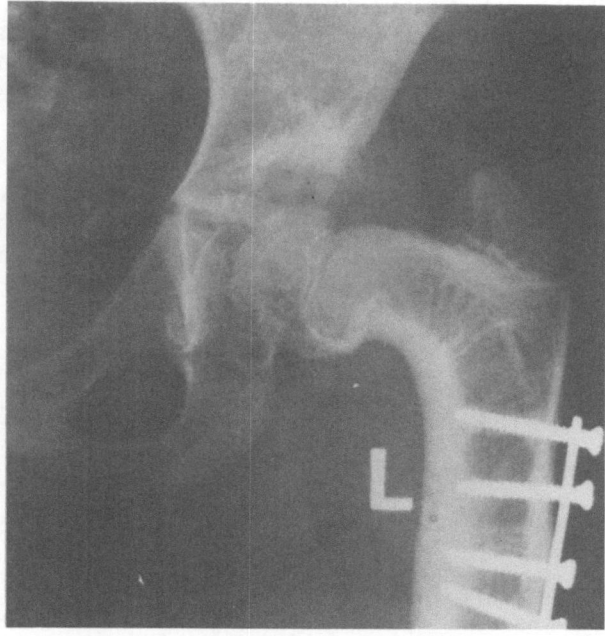

Fig. 5.63. Varus, as shown here, with sclerosis of the calcar does not improve because it is a growth disturbance. For some reason it does not get any worse. Anteversion does not recur in the presence of this deformity

a simple bending of the neck, which will correct itself spontaneously and for which active treatment is contraindicated. Spontaneous bending of the neck may occur in children over the age of 3 years at the time of treatment with bilateral dislocations. If at the end of treatment there is some undue stiffness of the hips adduction may develop owing to bending at the femoral necks instead of at the hip joints (Fig. 5.64).

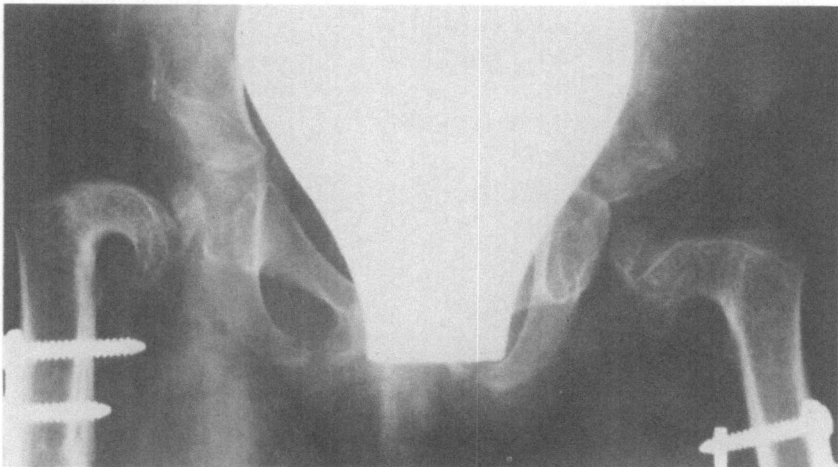

Fig. 5.64. Varus which is due to bending, as seen in both these hips, is not a growth deformity and will correct spontaneously without treatment

Without any treatment the deformity steadily improved over a period of 5 years until normal neck-shaft angles were achieved with satisfactory acetabular development (Fig. 5.65). It is possible to differentiate between these two conditions by the appearance on the radiograph of an area of sclerosis on the underside of the femoral neck when there is a growth deformity (Fig. 5.63).

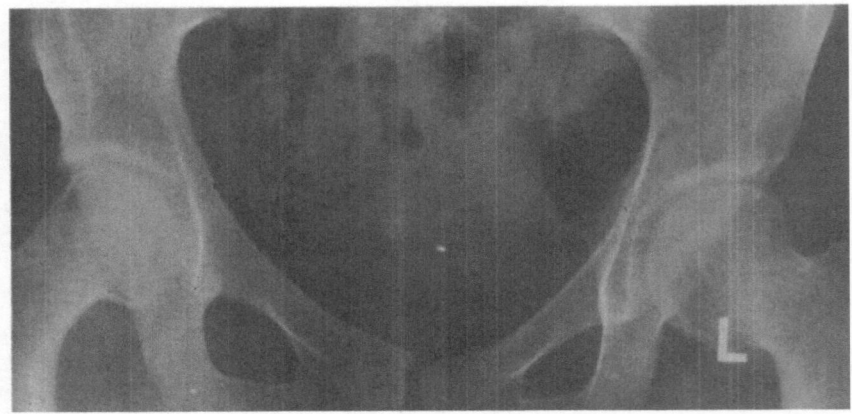

Fig. 5.65. Thirteen years after the radiograph shown in Fig. 5.64 was taken, the neck-shaft angles are normal

REFERENCES

Harris NH, Lloyd-Roberts GC, Gallien R (1975) Acetabular development in congenital dislocation of the hip. J Bone Joint Surg [Br] 57:46
Haas J (1948) Congenital dislocation of the hip. Thomas, Springfield
O'Malley AG (1963) The influence of the flexor and adductor muscles on the hip joint. Clin Orthop 31:73
Somerville EW (1974) The nature of the congenitally dislocated hip. Proc R Soc Med 67:1169
Trueta J (1957) The normal vascular anatomy of the human femoral head during growth. J Bone Joint Surg [Br] 39:358

6 Operations on the Pelvis

The foregoing chapters in this book have been devoted to demonstrating how the development of the acetabulum is dependent on the mechanics of the joint and that if concentric movement of the femoral head in the acetabulum can be achieved the acetabulum will develop satisfactorily, often in the most unlikely cases. It is logical that if the acetabulum can be made to develop normally without any alteration to its shape or direction this is preferable to carrying out some plastic procedure on the joint. Nevertheless, when such damage has been done to the acetabulum, either by time or trauma, that it is too difficult to restore concentric movement it may become necessary to alter the shape or direction of the acetabulum.

Three types of operation have been used for this purpose: (1) the innominate osteotomy (Salter 1966); (2) the Pemberton osteotomy (Pemberton 1965); and (3) the Chiari osteotomy (Chiari 1955, 1974).

INNOMINATE OSTEOTOMY (SALTER)

In this operation the innominate bone is divided above the acetabulum. The lower fragment is pulled downwards and forwards so that the anterior lip of the acetabulum will form an actual bony barrier to the displacement of the femoral head anteriorly. This operation is combined with an anterior capsuloplasty and division of the psoas tendon. The displacement of the lower fragment is maintained by a wedge of bone cut from the iliac crest. Because this is often unstable it should be maintained in position with two Kirschner wires, and the hip is immobilised in plaster for 6–8 weeks until union is sound.

In the hands of a surgeon experienced in this type of surgery the operation gives very satisfactory results (Salter 1974). But it is an operation whose results can be unpredictable. If the lower fragment has been properly displaced it is observed in the postoperative radiograph that the obturator foramen on the side operated upon appears to have been substantially narrowed compared with the one on the other side. Unless this can be demonstrated there is no evidence that the direction of the acetabulum has been appreciably altered. All that has happened is that the ilium has been displaced upwards, as can sometimes be demonstrated by the obliquity of the iliac crests. This is more likely to happen if there has been extensive stripping of the muscles from the iliac crest. Such stripping of the muscles makes the division of the innominate bone very much easier, but it also makes the subsequent stability of the ilium dependent entirely on the re-attachment of the muscles over the iliac crest, from which a graft will already have been removed. But even in cases where it is obvious that the ilium has been displaced upwards and the change in the direction of the acetabulum is minimal an excellent result will often be obtained provided a good capsulorrhaphy has been performed. This emphasises the importance of the division of the psoas tendon, which removes the deforming force, and of the capsulorrhaphy, which provides stability.

A child aged 3 years was found to have a dislocated hip. The dislocation was reduced by traction, and an innominate osteotomy was performed without division of the psoas tendon or a capsulorrhaphy. After removal of the plaster the hip rapidly became redisplaced (Fig. 6.1). Reduction was achieved easily by simple medial rotation, and this was maintained by a high femoral osteotomy with lateral rotation and varus (Fig. 6.2); the hip has since continued to develop satisfactorily, as was seen 2 years later (Fig. 6.3).

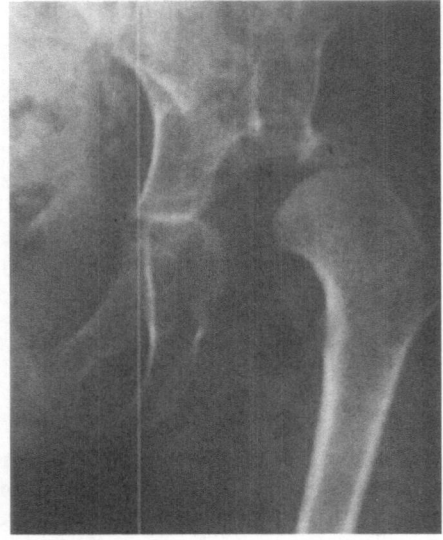

Fig. 6.1. Hip showing redisplacement after innominate osteotomy in which neither a capsulorrhaphy nor division of the psoas was performed

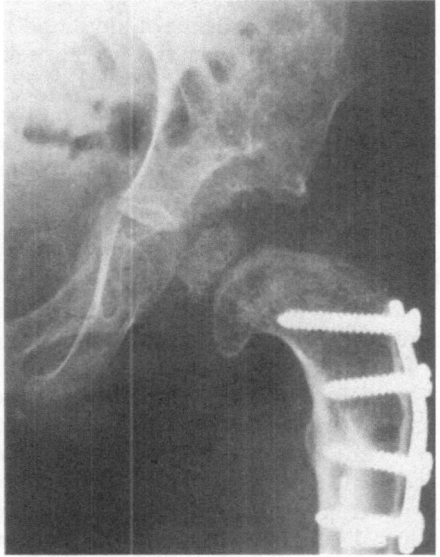

Fig. 6.2. The same hip as in Fig. 6.1, seen 7 months after high femoral osteotomy with 70° of rotation and 15° of varus

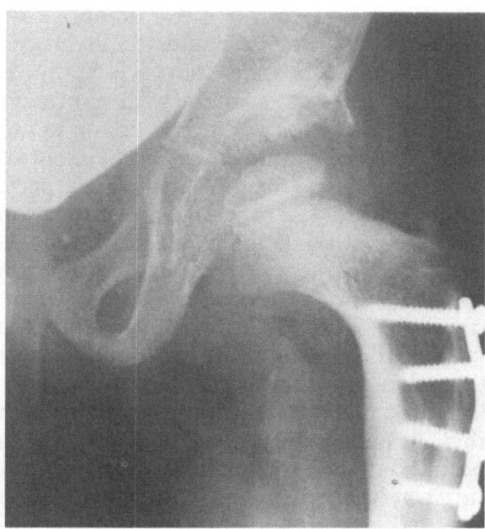

Fig. 6.3. Two-and-a-half years later the position of the hip seen in Fig. 6.2 is now stable

A further difficulty with this operation is that if the acetabulum is actually deformed the head of the femur will not fit congruously into it before the operation, and because the shape of the acetabulum is not altered there will still be incongruity afterwards, though if the child is young enough remodelling will gradually take place.

THE PEMBERTON OSTEOTOMY

It is for these reasons that in this series of cases, when a pelvic reconstruction operation has been required a Pemberton type of osteotomy, which is rather more versatile, has been preferred. The operation has been carried out through a slightly oblique transverse incision about 1 in. below the anterior superior iliac spine and about 3 in. in length. The cartilaginous apophysis is split down the middle from the anterior superior iliac spine posteriorly for 2–3 in. and the two halves with the attached muscles are reflected subperiosteally to expose the medial and lateral surfaces of the ilium anteriorly. Medially the subperiosteal separation is carried posteriorly to the sciatic notch, into which a bone lever is placed, and the separation is extended inferiorly to expose the triradiate cartilage. The rectus muscle with its reflected head is identified and the capsule defined. This will be difficult if the operation is being performed as a salvage procedure, because there will often be distortion of the anatomy and much scarring. Subperiosteal separation is then carried out above the acetabulum sufficiently to allow the introduction of a bone lever into the sciatic notch from the outer side; the tip of this bone lever will encounter the tip of the one on the medial side. A wedge graft is removed from the iliac crest with a saw to prevent crushing or splitting. This is done before the osteotomy so that the pelvis will be firm to cut. The base of the wedge will usually be about ¾ in., though in the bigger child it may have to be a little larger. The direction of the displacement of the acetabular roof will be determined by the plane of the osteotomy. The nearer this plane is to the horizontal, the more the displacement will be anterior; and the more oblique the plane of osteotomy the more lateral the displacement will be. Generally the osteotomy will be so aligned that the displacement will be about 45°. The osteotomy is started about ½ in. above the estimated lip of the acetabulum. If the procedure follows a capsulorrhaphy, for which the joint will have been opened, the positioning of the osteotomy will be much easier.

The initial cut is made with a broad straight osteotome aimed in an exactly posterior direction and this is driven in until it is estimated that it is well clear of the joint. The osteotome is then directed inferiorly towards the sciatic notch just above the triradiate cartilage. This is made easier and safer if an osteotome curved in its length is used. If a broad osteotome is used its progress can be observed under direct vision on both the medial and lateral aspects of the pelvis, and when it appears that it has reached the posterior cortex it is levered firmly downwards. If a greenstick fracture is not produced then it is driven in rather further until the cortex can be fractured easily. The fracture is not displaced. The acetabular roof is rotated forwards and laterally by the introduction of a broad flat instrument placed well back in the osteotomy and forcibly rotated in such a way as to rotate the roof forwards and laterally; this will then allow room for the introduction of the wedge anteriorly. After this has been driven home carefully with a punch, it will be found that it is so firmly jammed that no form of internal fixation is necessary. When the operation is done in this way there is no question of the ilium being pushed up. The osteotomy must always be done with the head of the femur in the acetabulum so that if there is deformity of the acetabular roof it will be moulded to the head and produce a congruous joint (Figs. 6.4–6.6).

A great advantage of this operation is its versatility. It is not always necessary or desirable to carry the osteotomy through the full thickness of the pelvis. Where the coverage of the head is not quite sufficient to ensure longevity of the joint (Fig. 6.7) the position can be corrected quite easily by using the same technique, with the minor modification that the osteotomy does not quite reach the inner cortex (Fig. 6.8); but the roof can be moulded down over the femoral head to provide better coverage (Fig. 6.9).

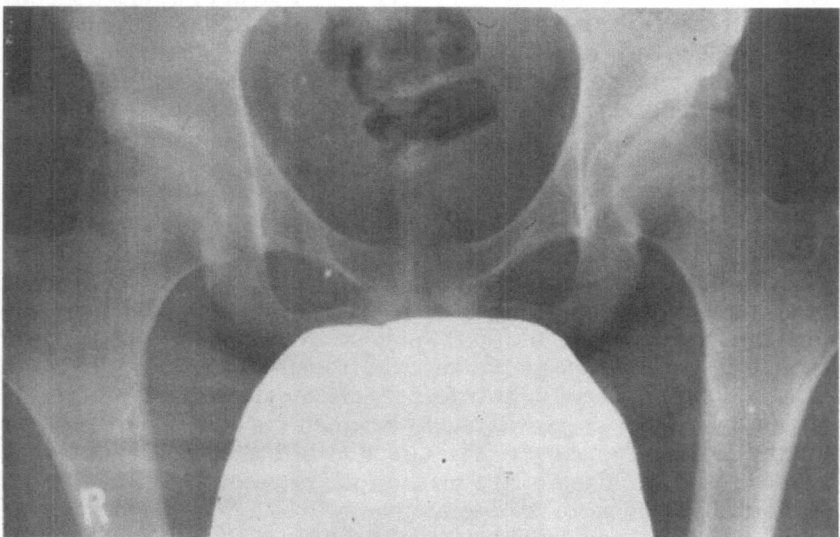

Fig. 6.4. Dysplasia of the hips in boy of 16. There is no displacement but he is already complaining of pain

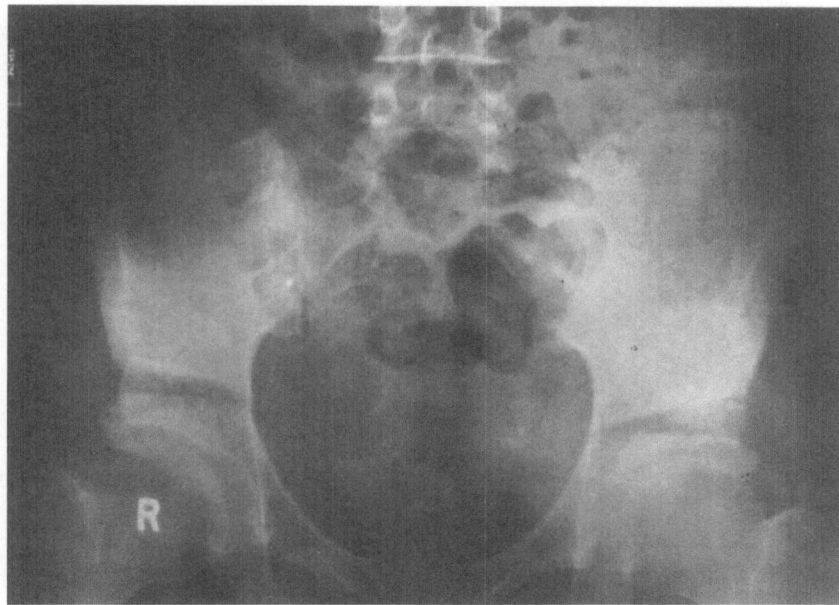

Fig. 6.5. Same hip as in Fig. 6.4, following pelvic osteotomy in which the acetabular roofs were moulded over the femoral heads

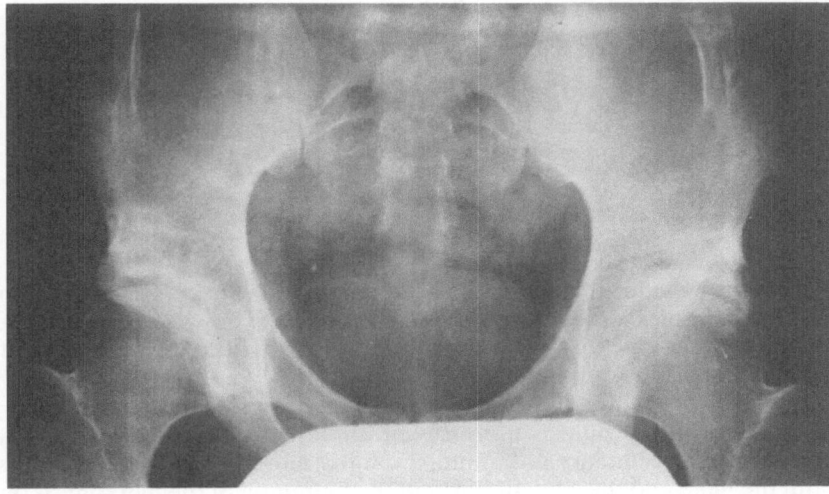

Fig. 6.6. The same hips as in Figs. 6.4 and 6.5, seen 3 years later

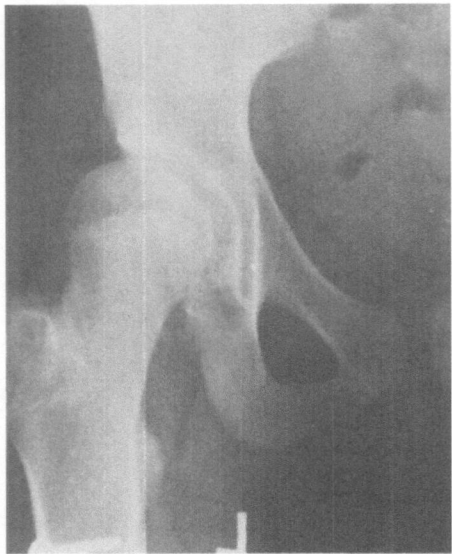

Fig. 6.7. Previously treated bilateral dislocations. The left femoral head is not well covered and there is perhaps a very minimal degree of subluxation

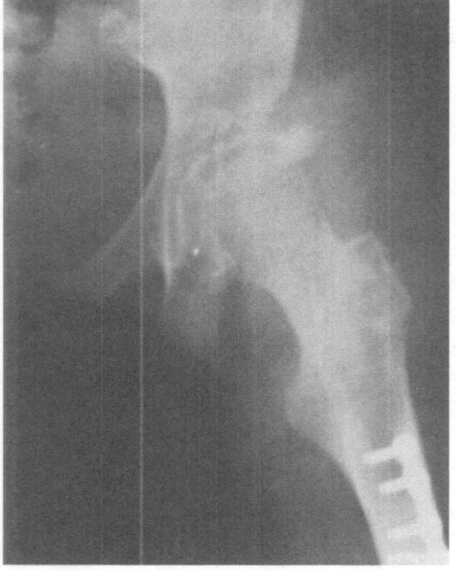

Fig. 6.8. The same hip as in Fig. 6.7, immediately after osteotomy

There is no value in making the acetabulum too capacious. The evidence suggests that too deep an acetabulum providing too much cover will lead to early degenerative changes just as quickly as an acetabulum which is a little too shallow, and sometimes more quickly. The aim must be to get it just right.

Figure 6.10 shows the severely dislocated hips in a child aged 3 years. The dislocation on the right is more severe than the one on the left, as shown by the presence of a secondary acetabulum and the more severely retarded ossification in both the head and the acetabulum and the flattening of the metaphysis on the medial side suggesting damage to the blood supply to the medial side of the head. After

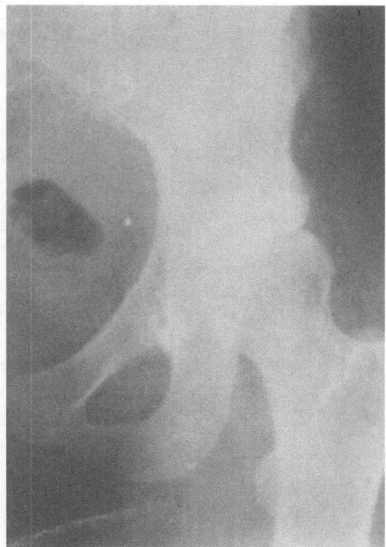

Fig. 6.9. The same hip as in Figs. 6.7 and 6.8, seen 3 years later

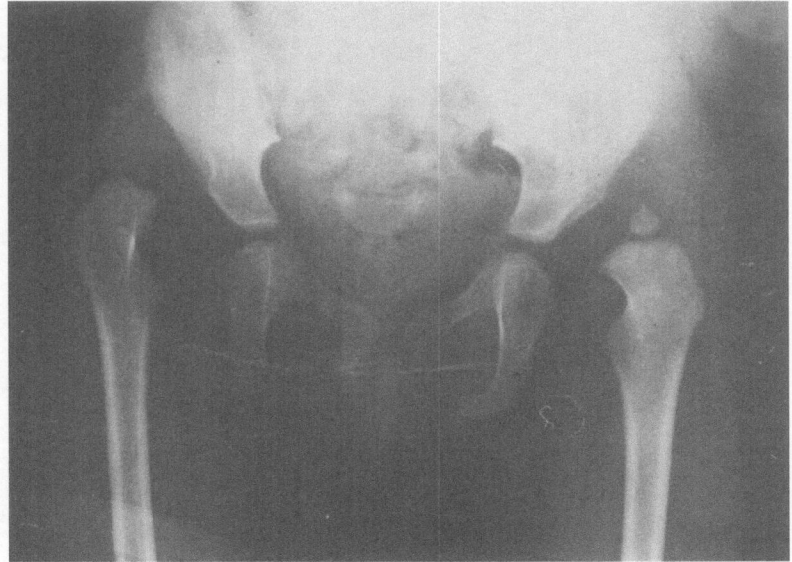

Fig. 6.10. Bilateral dislocations. The right is worse than the left, as can be seen from the reduced ossification and evidence of pressure on the medial side of the head and neck

routine treatment on both sides (Fig. 6.11) it appears that the left hip is developing satisfactorily, but on the right there is subluxation and the medial side of the head has not developed at all. An arthrogram (Fig. 6.12) shows that there is an actual defect of the cartilaginous lip of the acetabulum. This was corrected by turning down the lip of the acetabulum anterosuperiorly, superiorly, and posterosuperiorly to the depth of about ¾ in. (Fig. 6.13). Following this the head remained in the reduced position and

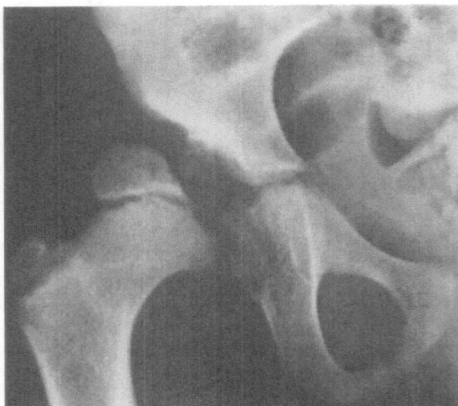

Fig. 6.11. Four years later, while the left hip shown in Fig. 6.10 has developed well, the right hip is displaced and the medial side of the femoral head has never developed

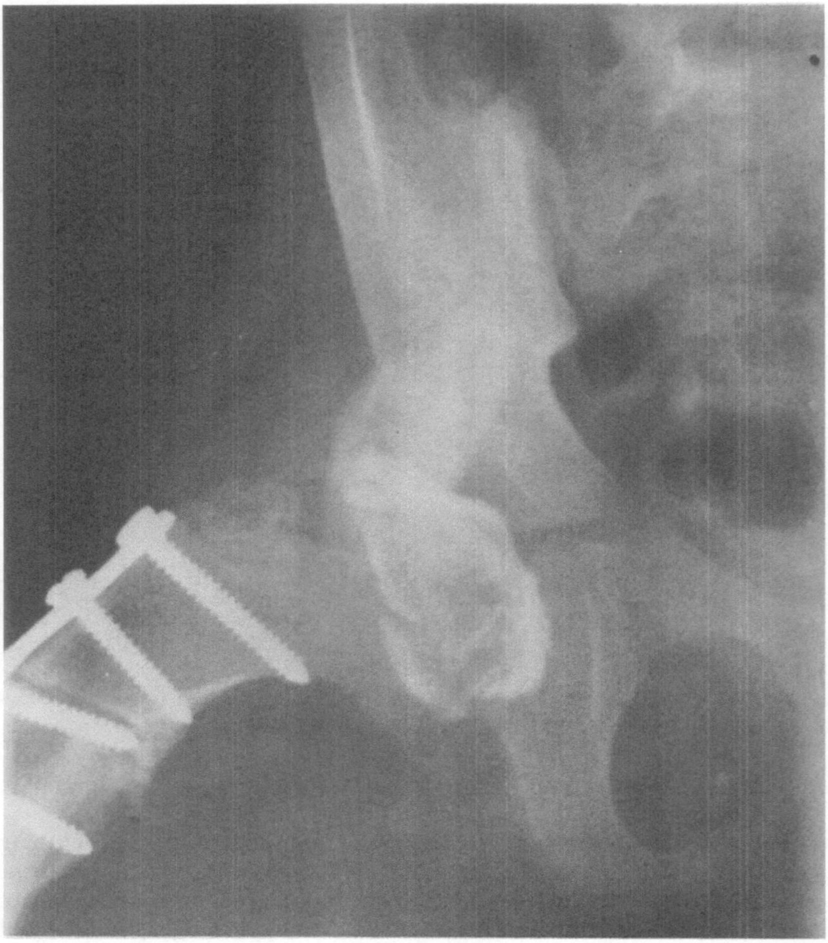

Fig. 6.12. Same patient as in Figs. 6.10 and 6.11. The arthrogram shows a defect in the cartilaginous lip of the acetabulum

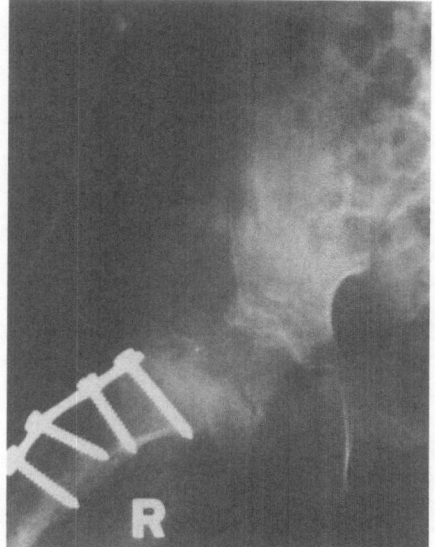

Fig. 6.13. Same patient as in Figs. 6.10–6.12, immediately following lowering of the lip of the acetabulum

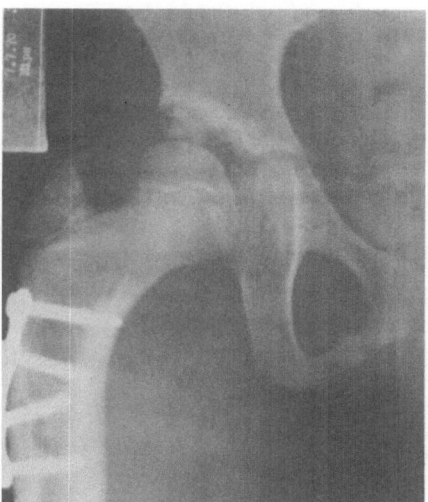

Fig. 6.14. Two years later, the position of the hip shown in Figs. 6.10–6.13 has been maintained and ossification is taking place in the roof of the acetabulum

ossification can be seen developing in the cartilaginous roof of the acetabulum (Fig. 6.14). Five years later the position had been maintained, and even though the stigma in the femoral head remains the acetabulum is well shaped and there is adequate coverage of the head (Fig. 6.15).

In both these types of operation the object is to restore the normal relationship between the femoral head and the acetabulum and to provide stability and concentricity of movement so that normal development of the joint can be resumed. But sometimes the deformity of the joint is such that this is no longer possible.

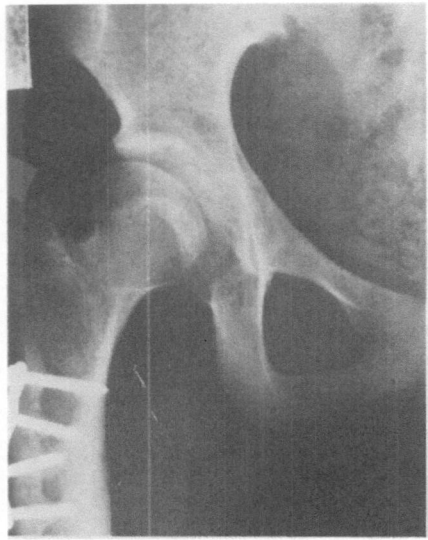

Fig. 6.15. Five years later the position of the hip shown in Figs. 6.10–6.14 is well maintained and the hip is growing well

THE CHIARI OSTEOTOMY

The operation known as the Chiari osteotomy was developed to deal with the cases described at the end of the last section (Fig. 6.16). The operation is essentially one for the older child, i.e., 7 years of age or older (Colton 1972), but on one occasion in this series the operation was carried out on a child of 4, with a remarkably satisfactory result. There are three criteria which indicate the necessity for operation. The child is complaining of pain; there is a severe limp; or there is radiological evidence of

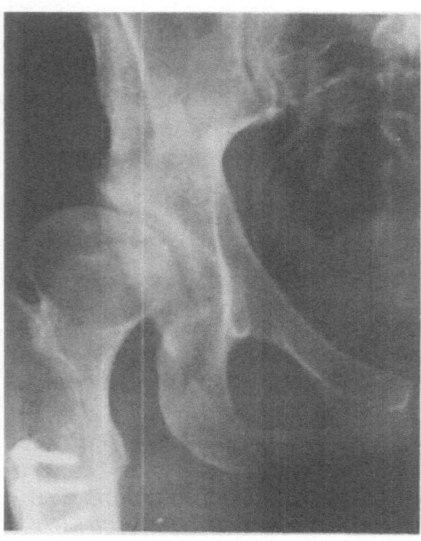

Fig. 6.16. Poor result following treatment for a congenitally dislocated hip in a girl now aged 27

increasing displacement. This last is perhaps the most important of all. Displacement will often increase gradually without any obvious change in signs or symptoms, and if this is allowed to happen the wall of the pelvis will become increasingly thinned until a point is reached when the operation is not possible because adequate displacement is not practicable. At a later date it will also be extremely difficult to perform an arthrodesis or, should it be considered wise, to introduce a total hip replacement. The radiological diagnosis of thinning is often very misleading because in the antero-posterior radiograph the pelvic wall is seen obliquely, completely disguising the true thickness.

The operation has been carried out through a straight incision similar to that used for a Pemberton osteotomy, and if the apophysis is still cartilaginous it is split in the same way, with as little separation of the muscle from the iliac crest as possible. On the outer side the muscle is reflected subperiosteally down to the capsule of the joint, which is cleared of fat until its attachment to the pelvis can be clearly demarcated. The subperiosteal reflection is then carried posteriorly to the sciatic notch into which a broad bone lever is placed. Care must be taken to ensure that the bone lever is placed between the periosteum and the bone, so that the important structures in the notch are protected from damage. On the inner side of the pelvis the periosteal stripping is only sufficient to allow the introduction of the bone lever into the notch, where it will come into contact with the other one.

The site and direction of the osteotomy must be selected with great care and it is best carried out under radiological control (Fig. 6.17). A thin Steinmann's pin is introduced at what is estimated to be 3 mm above the bony lip of the acetabulum. This position should not be ascertained by opening the capsule. The pin is driven through the pelvis in a slightly upward direction towards just below the sacro-iliac joint. The position is confirmed radiologically. The line of the osteotomy is then marked out on the outer side of the pelvis. It must be slightly curved upwards, starting low anteriorly, rising in the middle, and becoming low again posteriorly. This curve cannot possibly make the acetabulum congruous with the femoral head, but it will prevent anterior or posterior slipping of one fragment on the other. Should such displacement occur it can present a considerable problem in instability. Also, the downward curvature posteriorly will help to prevent the extension of the osteotomy upwards into the sacro-iliac joint, which will make medial displacement very difficult.

In cutting during the osteotomy it is wise to retain the pin in position for as long as possible to indicate the direction required. Two $\frac{1}{2}$ in. osteotomes are used rather than one broad one. The first one is driven part way through the bone anteriorly and the second one immediately posterior to it, the first one being used as a guide for the second. After that they leap-frog each other round to the sciatic notch. Each osteotome is only driven half-way through the bone. The osteotomes are then used again in the same way, this time being driven right through the bone either under direct vision, or, if this is not possible, onto a finger introduced inside the pelvis. The cortex posteriorly in the sciatic notch is the most difficult part to divide; it is hard, inaccessible, and close to important structures. This cortex must be divided completely, because if it is not hingeing will occur instead of displacement. Probably the best way of dividing this cortex is by introducing a broad osteotome curved in its length anteriorly along the line of the osteotomy down to the intact cortex posteriorly, which can then be divided with a sharp blow. The important structures are protected either by the bone levers or, preferably, by a swab passed through the notch. This technique also reduces the risk of the osteotomy extending up into the sacro-iliac joint.

It has been suggested that the posterior cortex can be divided more easily with a Gigli saw; but the use of this instrument will necessitate too much stripping of the

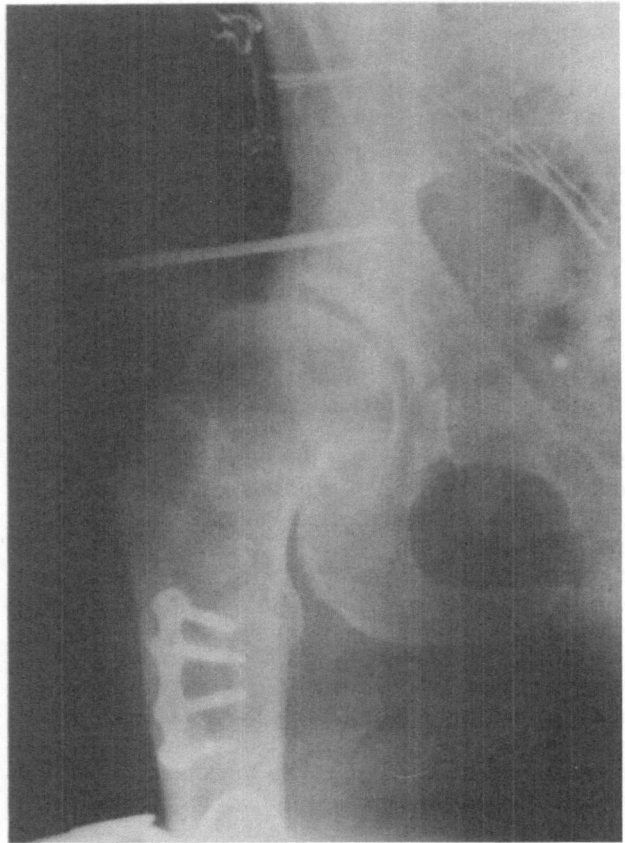

Fig. 6.17. Steinmann pin used as a marker to determine the correct level. The osteotomy will be carried out between the pin and the lip of the acetabulum. The direction is good

muscles. This often causes the osteotomy to become unstable and must be avoided.

The displacement is most satisfacorily accomplished from within the pelvis, rather than by pressure exerted on the femur from the outside. A 1 in. osteotome is introduced into the osteotomy in its length and is firmly rotated in such a way that the lower fragment is displaced medially to rather more than half the width of the pelvic wall. If the muscle stripping has been minimal the position will be stable and internal fixation will not be necessary (Fig. 6.18). The muscles are sutured back in position and the wound is closed. The hip is immobilised in a plaster spica in about 20° of abduction for 8 weeks, when non-weight-bearing mobilisation is started. The leg should not be immobilised in wide abduction because in this position there is a real risk of complete medial displacement, which will prolong the time taken for union (Figs. 6.19 and 6.20).

The early results of this operation have sometimes been disappointing. Pain has often been a nuisance and may on occasions persist for a year or more, but with very few exceptions it has eventually gone. In the absence of any obvious cause for this it is most likely that sound bony union has taken longer than was expected, and even longer than the radiological appearance had suggested. In the long term, however, the results have been most satisfactory (Figs. 6.21 and 6.22).

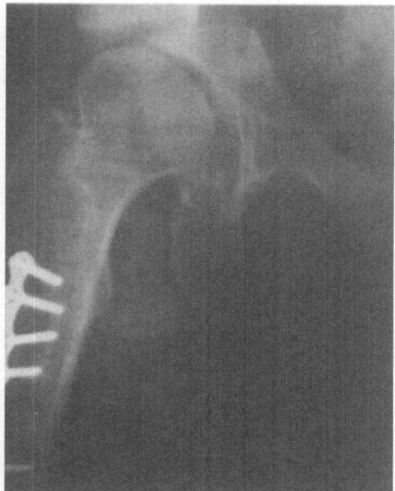

Fig. 6.18. Osteotomy, as carried out following
determination of the correct level as shown in Fig. 6.17

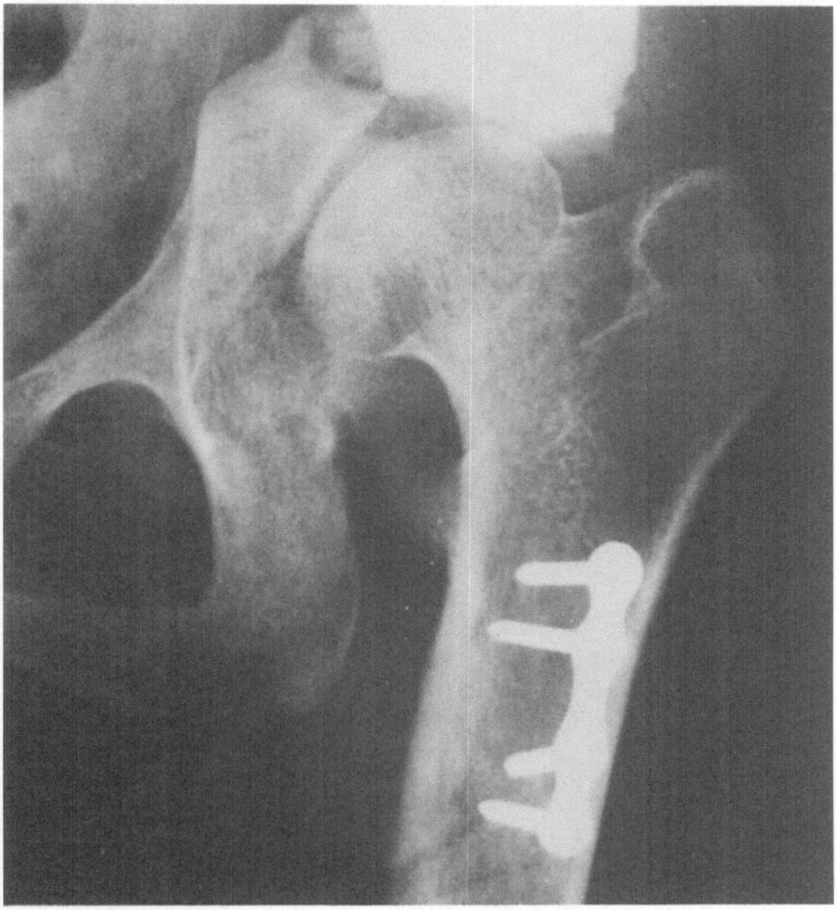

Fig. 6.19. Full-thickness displacement

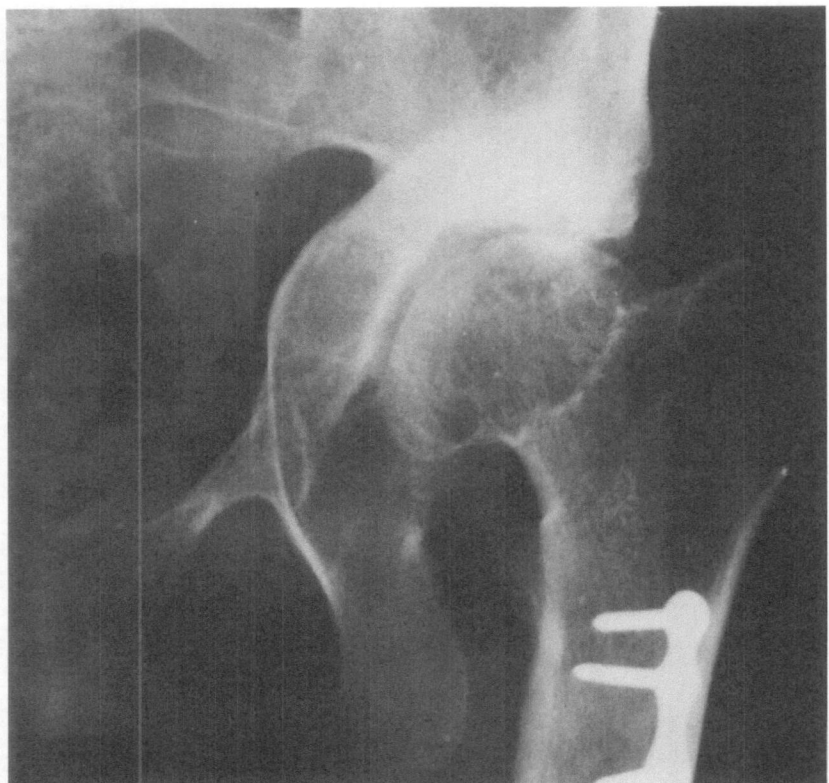

Fig. 6.20. The final result of the displacement shown in Fig. 6.19 was good, but it took 18 months to unite. This radiograph was taken more than 6 years after operation

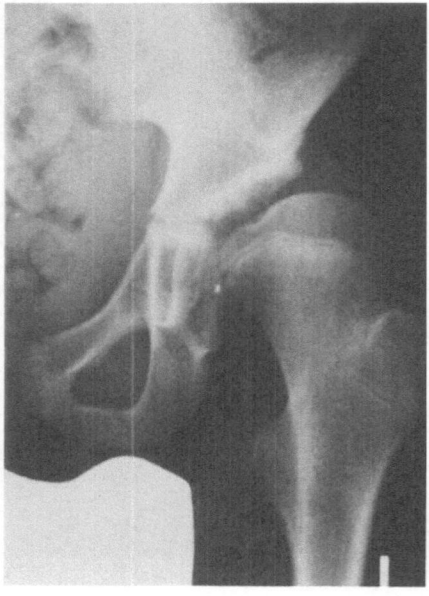

Fig. 6.21. Untreated displacement already causing pain in a boy of 13

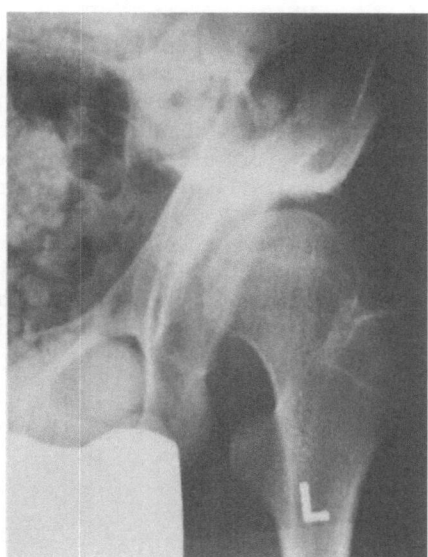

Fig. 6.22. Three years after a Chiari osteotomy, full function has been restored to the displaced hip shown in Fig. 6.22. It is interesting that the dew-drop, which was broad, is now narrow

Another cause of pain and stiffness which is occasionally encountered appears to be cartilage necrosis. This has only been seen in those hips in which the siting of the osteotomy has appeared to be perfect or perhaps too near the lip. It has not been seen in those hips in which the osteotomy has left a slight step, though this step should not be more than minimal. In these cases gentle non-weight-bearing mobilisation for many months with the patient kept strictly on crutches has allowed the condition to resolve. In the case of a girl aged 9 years with bilateral severe subluxations associated with some degree of spasticity (Fig. 6.23) traction was applied to pull the head down

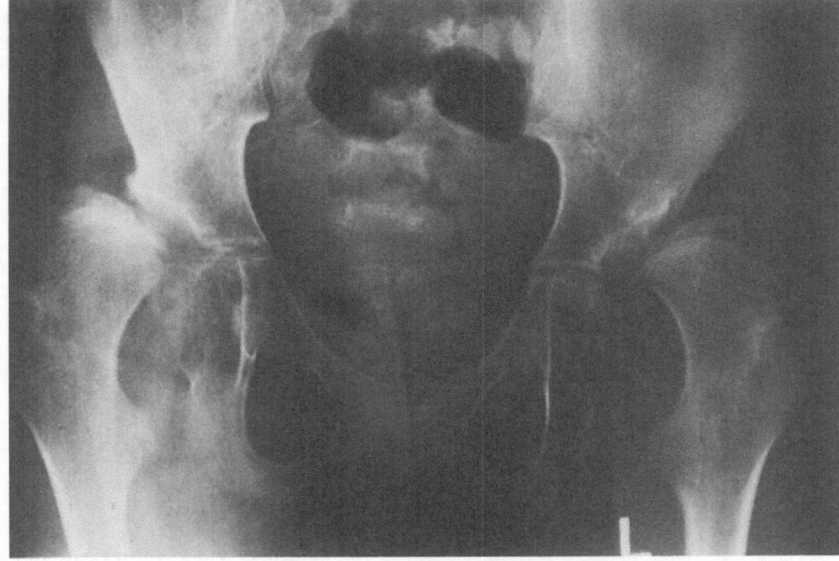

Fig. 6.23. Displacement with spasticity in a girl aged 9. This was causing great pain in the right hip

after an adductor tenotomy. The osteotomy was performed through the bony lip and appeared to be excellent, but the hip became stiff and painful and it became apparent that cartilage necrosis had developed. Because of the risk of producing two stiff hips it was not possible to operate on the other hip until it was too late. For about 3 years the untreated hip remained the better of the two. The treated hip then improved and developed a very useful range of movement without pain and became by far the better of the two (Fig. 6.24). Except in cases such as this, stiffness has not presented a problem.

Sometimes as a result of faulty technique the osteotomy is performed too high, leaving a considerable gap (Fig. 6.25). In spite of this the symptoms in one patient were relieved for 2 years, after which pain and aching returned as before. In such a case the gap can be filled with a full-thickness piece of ilium, taking care that when the

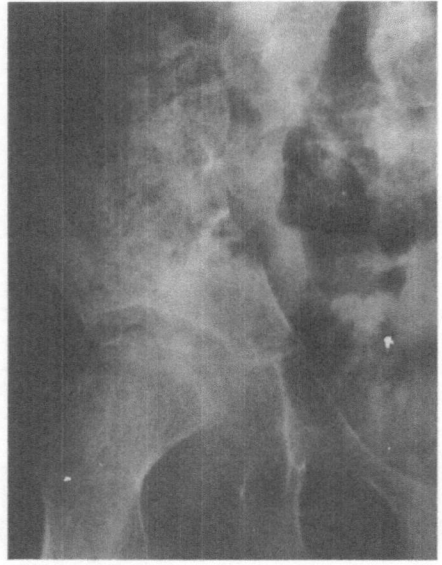

Fig. 6.24. A satisfactory result was eventually achieved in the displaced hip shown in Fig. 6.23, as seen 5 years later, although it was very slow in developing

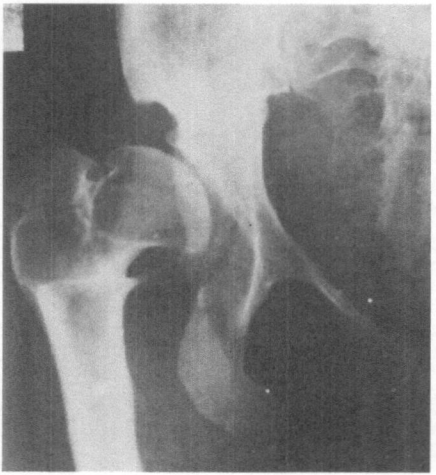

Fig. 6.25. Unsatisfactory osteotomy done too high, which gave only temporary relief

bone surfaces are being prepared the capsule is not damaged (Fig. 6.26). In the case illustrated the result has been most satisfactory for 5 years, during which time the patient has worked as a school teacher and has given birth to a child.

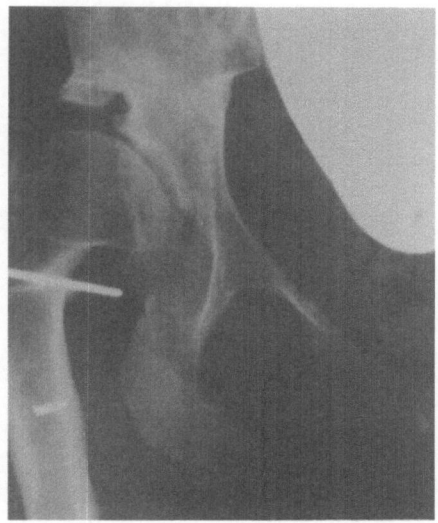

Fig. 6.26. Stability of the hip shown in Fig. 6.25 has been improved by introduction of a piece of ilium into the gap

The persistence of a limp after the operation has been rather disappointing, though it has been noted many times that what appeared to be a persistent limp has, like pain, improved remarkably with time. In cases where the limp has not improved, transfer of the greater trochanter downwards may be helpful. When the operation is performed for a limp it is wise to do this routinely.

Age does not seem to have had any particular effect on the result, but it is better not to do the operation in a patient under the age of 7. The oldest patient in this series was 27, and the operation was not noticeably more difficult than in the younger patients. Postoperative recovery is probably rather quicker in the young patients, though the difference has not been marked. Probably the ideal age range is 7–16 years.

REFERENCES

Chiari K (1955) Ergebnisse mit der Beckenosteotomie als Pfannendachplastik. Z Orthop 87:14
Chiari K (1974) Medial displacement osteotomy. Clin Orthop 98:35
Colton CL (1972) Chiari osteotomy for acetabular dysplasia in young subjects. J Bone Joint Surg [Br] 54:579
Pemberton PA (1965) Pericapsular osteotomy of the ilium in congenital dislocation and subluxation of the hip. J Bone Joint Surg [Am] 47:65
Salter RB (1966) Role of innominate osteotomy in the treatment of congenital dislocation and subluxation in the older child. J Bone Joint Surg [Am] 48:1413
Salter RB (1974) 15 years' experience with innominate osteotomy in the treatment of congenital dislocation and subluxation of the hip. Clin Orthop 98:72

7 Some Iatrogenic Problems

Some of the problems resulting from either faulty or misguided treatment have already been described and ways of treating them discussed. But there are two other problems which must be recognised because of the great difficulties which will inevitably result if they are not diagnosed at once. These are (1) fracture of the femur; and (2) extreme anteversion.

FRACTURE OF THE FEMUR

Fracture of the femur has been seen only in the lower quarter of the shaft in the supracondylar region. Most commonly it is seen in the first few days after mobilisation has started. The child is restless and miserable, and is not unnaturally unwilling to start mobilising. Examination will show a painful swelling just above the knee and slight forward bowing of the femur at this point. A radiograph clearly shows the presence of a greenstick fracture. It is rare for the angulation to be sufficient to require correction, but if it has been missed for several days this may be required. The fracture occurs spontaneously without any evidence of trauma, and is due to decalcification consequent upon immobilisation in plaster. The incidence of such fractures has been very low and there has been no evidence to suggest that they are more likely to occur in those children in whom for some reason the immobilisation has been rather longer than routinely expected.

Treatment has presented no problems. The knee is immobilised in a long well-fitting plaster cylinder for 3 weeks, after which mobilisation may be restarted. In one child who was sent home to mobilise instead of staying in hospital for the first 10 days deformity developed and the fracture united with deformity. This had to be corrected by a supracondylar osteotomy. Otherwise no complications have been encountered from this minor misfortune.

The second type of fracture, which has been encountered on three occasions, may lead to far more serious consequences.

This fracture has again been seen only in the lowest quarter of the femur. It has occurred during application of the plaster after excision of the limbus or open reduction (Fig. 7.1). It may be very difficult to detect that a fracture has occurred; there may have been no more than a slight click which can easily pass undetected, and it is possible that the instability will also pass undetected. The danger of this fracture is that all control of rotation is immediately lost, so that the surgeon may be under the impression that the hip is fully medially rotated, whereas it will only be the leg below the fracture. The upper part of the femur will not be medially rotated, with the result that the head of the femur is not in the acetabulum. The postoperative radiograph will show this displacement but not the cause (Fig. 7.2). In such circumstances it is wise to take a radiograph of the lower end of the femur (Fig. 7.3). Failure to diagnose

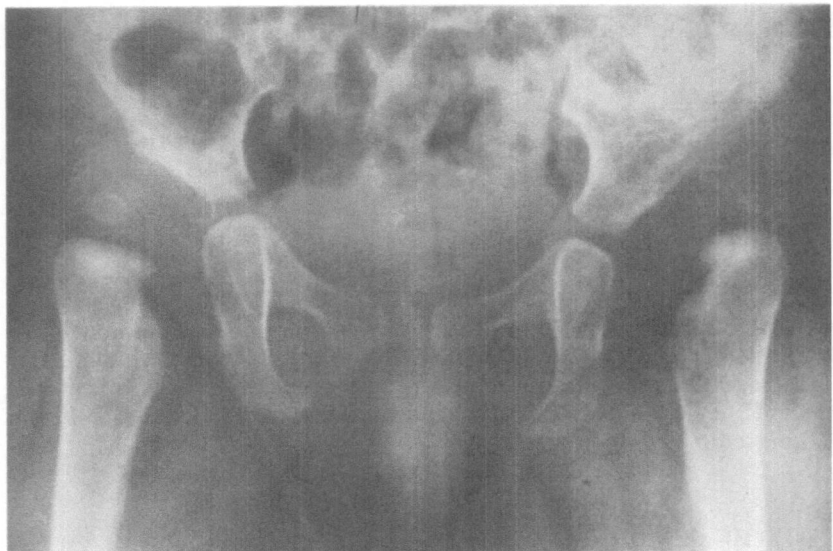

Fig. 7.1. Bilateral dislocations in a child aged 1 year. Attempts had previously been made elsewhere to reduce these dislocations, including an open operation on the left side when the child was 4 months old

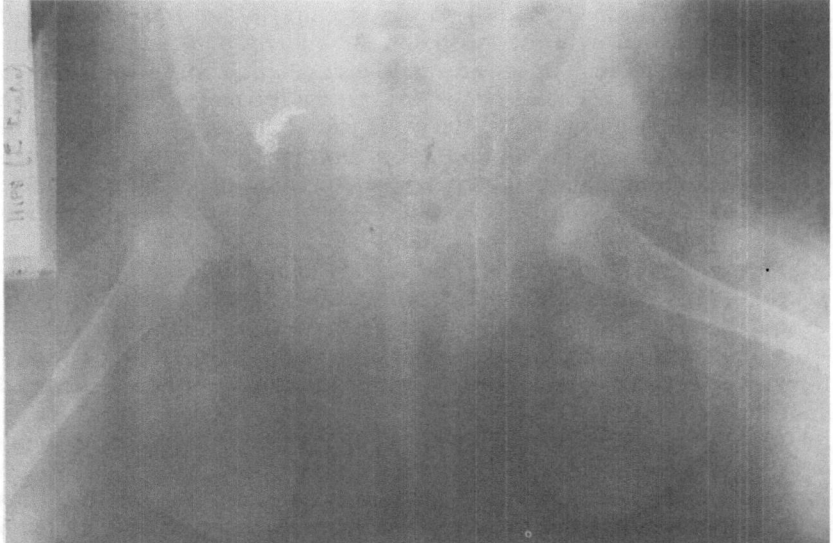

Fig. 7.2. Following bilateral excision of the limbuses in the patient shown in Fig. 7.1, the right hip is reduced but the left one is standing out and the upper end of the femur is not medially rotated

this fracture and to proceed to attempted manipulative or even open reduction of the hip will lead to obvious serious complications, which hardly need describing.

As soon as possible after the discovery of the fracture the upper fragment must be controlled by passing a Steinmann pin through the lower end of the upper fragment

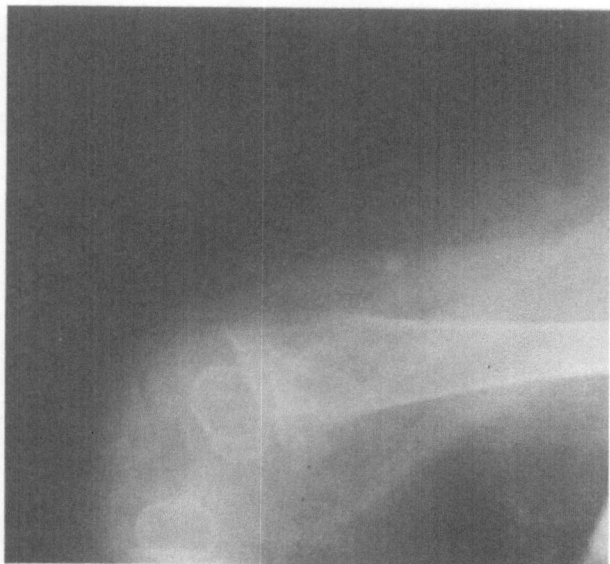

Fig. 7.3. A radiograph shows that the cause for the displacement in Fig. 7.2 is a fracture in the lower quarter of the femur

(Fig. 7.4). The upper fragment is rotated into full medial rotation by the pin and the lower leg is aligned correctly to it, including rotation, and a plaster spica including the pin is applied. The plaster is retained for 6 weeks, until the fracture is united beyond doubt, when a derotation ostetomy is carried out as previously described. Mobilisation is continued as in an uncomplicated case (Fig. 7.5).

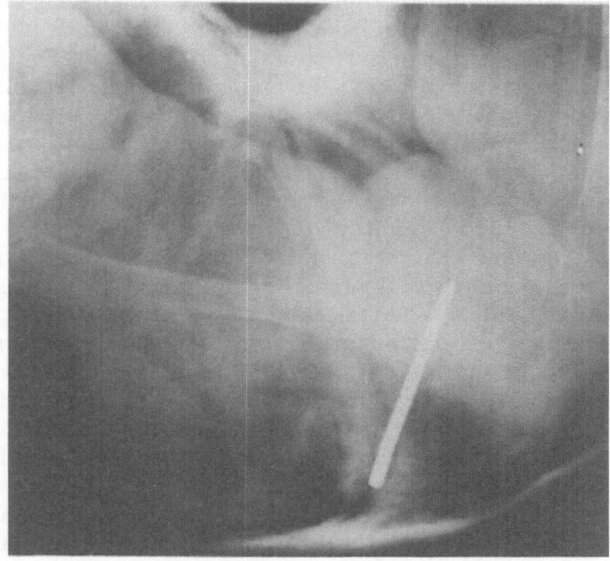

Fig. 7.4. The shaft of the femur above the fracture seen in Fig. 7.3 has been transfixed with a Steinmann pin. The femur can thus be medially rotated by the pin and the hip reduced

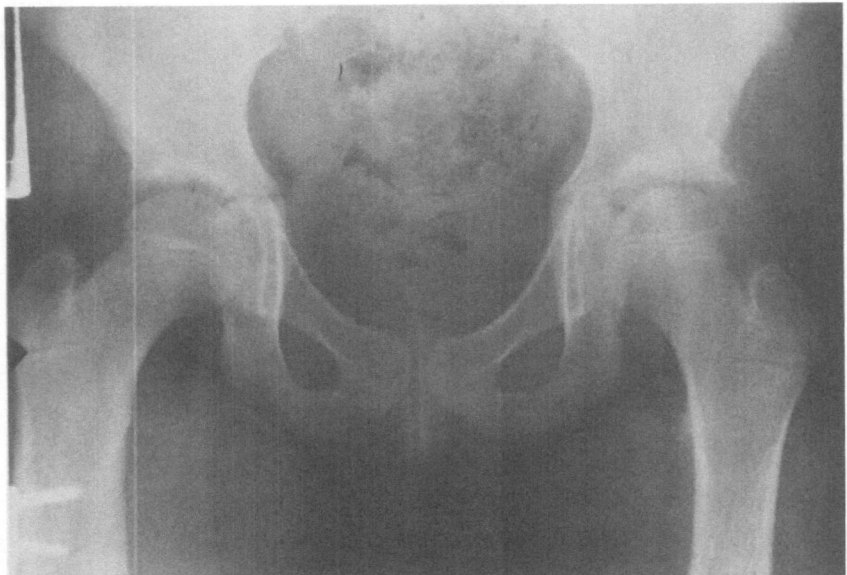

Fig. 7.5. The result of the fixation shown in Fig. 7.4, seen 9 years later, shows that both hips are satisfactory

EXTREME ANTEVERSION

As has already been described in Chapter 2, if the hip of a newborn child is put into the frog position without the displacement having been corrected, the femoral head will lie posterior to the acetabulum so that there will be continuous pressure on the posterior aspect of the femoral head (Fig. 2.9). This pressure may push the head and neck increasingly into anteversion. In some cases this will be as much as 160°–170°. When it is eventually discovered that the dislocation was never reduced great difficulty will be encountered in attempts to produce reduction. Any attempt at open reduction, when closed reduction has failed, will make matters even worse. When the joint is opened it will be found that it is not possible to rotate the femur far enough to replace the head in the joint.

Figure 7.6 shows the hips of a child at change of plaster holding the limbs in the frog position with the right hip displaced; the hip was kept unnoticed in this position for 9 months. When the child was seen at 18 months (Fig. 7.7) it was clear that there was very excessive anteversion. The head of the femur was almost reduced to the acetabulum on the frame and an open operation was carried out. It was only just possible to rotate the femur sufficiently to place the femoral head in the acetabulum with the femur rotated through about 140° and abducted 40°. The limb was splinted in plaster in this bizarre position. If further rotation had been necessary it would not have been possible to reduce the displacement. Subsequently a rotation osteotomy of 125° was performed and the final result was excellent (Fig. 7.8). It is interesting in this case to note that the left hip, which had never had anything wrong with it, shows definite evidence of injury to the growth plate, the result of the long period in plaster in the frog position.

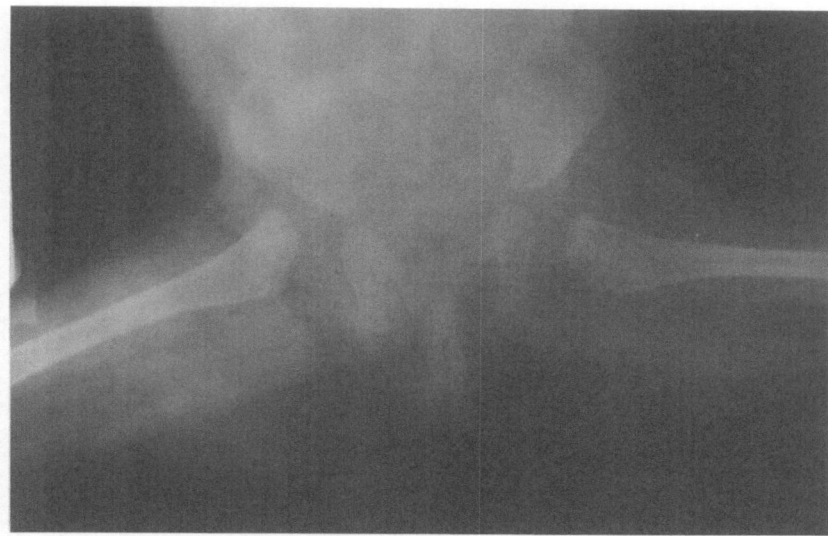

Fig. 7.6. The hips are in the frog position. The left hip is reduced but the right hip is dislocated

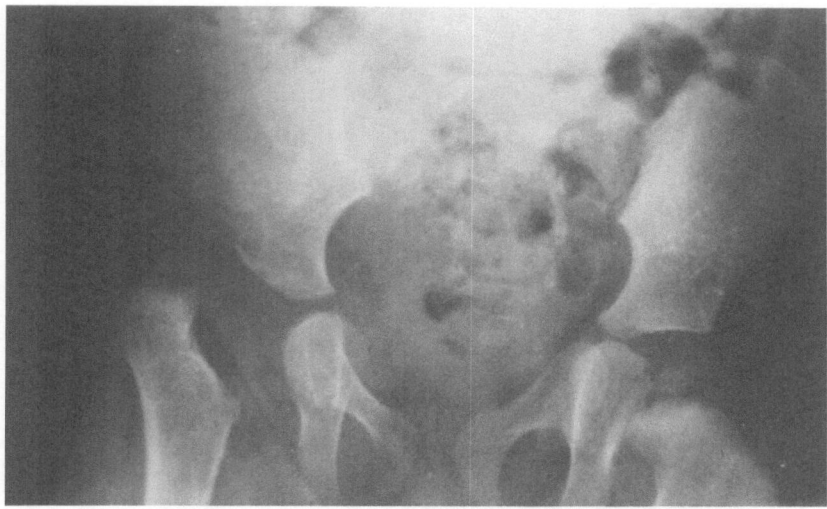

Fig. 7.7. At the age of 18 months there is obviously a very exaggerated degree of anteversion

In another child the dislocated hips diagnosed at birth were similarly mistreated. One hip was reduced but in the other the femoral head lay posterior to the acetabulum in the frog position for 6 months. At the age of 18 months the very severe degree of anteversion could be seen (Fig. 7.9). It was clear that it was not going to be possible to reduce this hip by any means because of this excessive anteversion. Without any attempt at reduction a rotation osteotomy of 90° was performed (Fig.

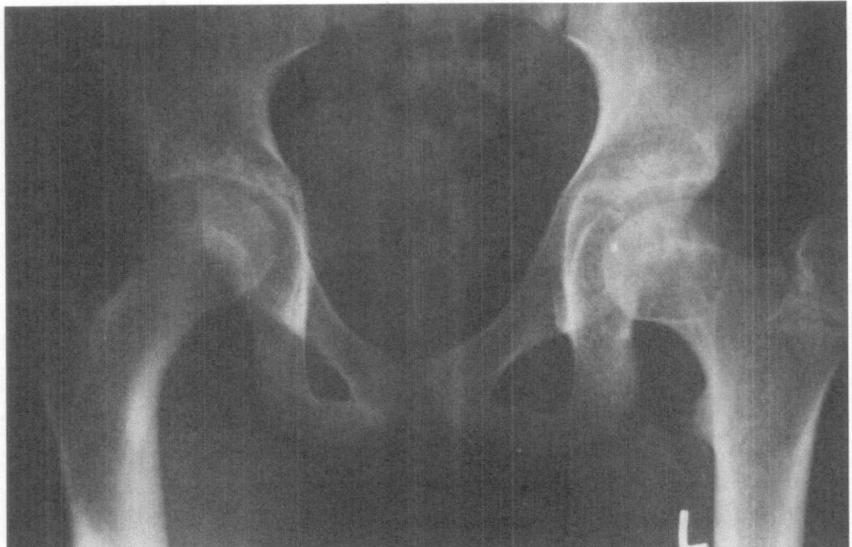

Fig. 7.8. Twelve years after treatment, the right hip is well reduced. The left hip, which was normal at birth, has developed a short neck and broad head due to damage to the growth plate at the initial treatment

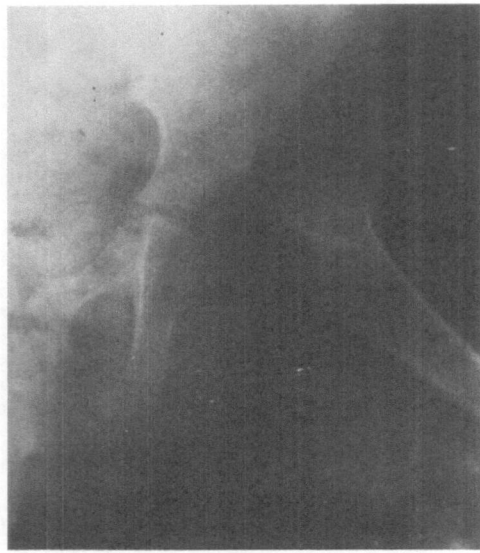

Fig. 7.9. A more severe case of excessive anteversion. This radiograph was taken with the left hip fully medially rotated

7.10). When the osteotomy was united the child was mobilised for 3 months until a reasonable range of movement had been achieved. Then routine treatment with frame reduction, arthrography, excision of the limbus and high femoral osteotomy with rotation of 70° was performed and subsequent mobilisation was uneventful. The position 10 years later (Fig. 7.11) shows that although there is still some varus in excess of normal the joint has developed satisfactorily, and apart from very slight limitation of abduction there was no limitation of movement.

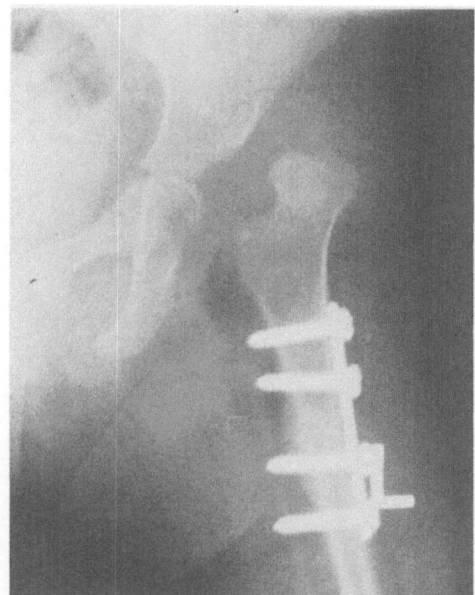

Fig. 7.10. Position following a rotation osteotomy of 90° without any attempt at reduction

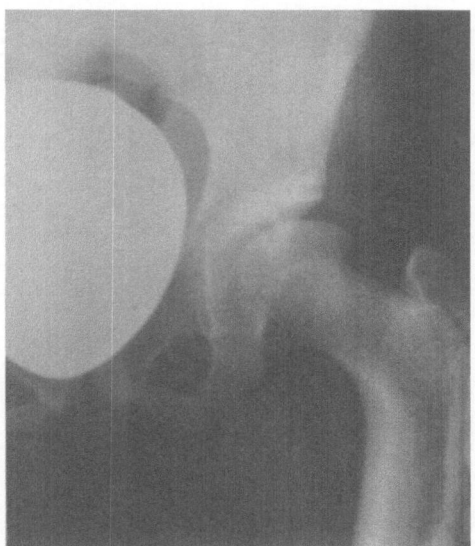

Fig. 7.11. Ten years after completion of treatment the hip is satisfactory, although the varus of the neck is persisting

Since our experience with these two hips four other hips have been treated in this way.

8 Perthes' Disease

Present knowledge suggests that Perthes' disease is primarily an ischaemia of the ossific nucleus of the head of the femur. The cause for this ischaemia has never been fully explained though there have been a number of hypotheses. Nor has there been any really convincing explanation as to why subluxation develops in a high proportion of cases. This subluxation has for long been overlooked because of the far more impressive changes taking place in the ossific nucleus. But it is becoming increasingly apparent that the correction of this subluxation providing total coverage of the femoral head is the most important factor in the treatment of this condition, and it is for this reason that a description of it is included here.

AETIOLOGY

In determining the underlying cause of Perthes' disease animal experiments have often been misleading, because while it is easy to produce avascular necrosis of the head of the femur it is extremely difficult to produce ischaemia of the ossific nucleus only. Some experiments, however, such as those described by Spivey and Parkes (1973) and Sanches et al. (1973), suggest that similar changes can be produced experimentally, though whether these can be translated into real life is difficult to say.

The onset is silent and the diagnosis is often not made until changes are well advanced; so that although the condition is commonly diagnosed between the ages of 4 and 10 years the actual onset must have been very much earlier; the reason why it is more common in boys than in girls is also unknown. In the great majority of cases there is no history of injury and it is exceptional to find anything suggesting a previous synovitis.

The ischaemia varies greatly both in its extent and in its intensity, both of which may be related to variations in the local anatomy. These anatomical variants may include increased vulnerability of the vessels in certain animals and in certain races, which may render them more or less prone to the disease.

The blood supply to the nucleus is by two and sometimes three routes. These routes have been well illustrated by the injection experiments of Trueta and Harrison (1953). The largest is a posterolateral leash of vessels supplying the anterolateral part of the nucleus. The others are a posteromedial leash, which is rather smaller and supplies the posteromedial portion, and a small inconstant vessel in the ligament of the femoral head (ligamentum teres), which is probably of little significance. The two main leashes are composed of three or four vessels each (Kemp 1973).

It is most commonly the anterolateral part of the nucleus which is involved (Fig. 8.1); this is supplied by the posterolateral leash which, lying as it does on the lateral aspect of the femoral neck, may in some people be vulnerable to being pinched

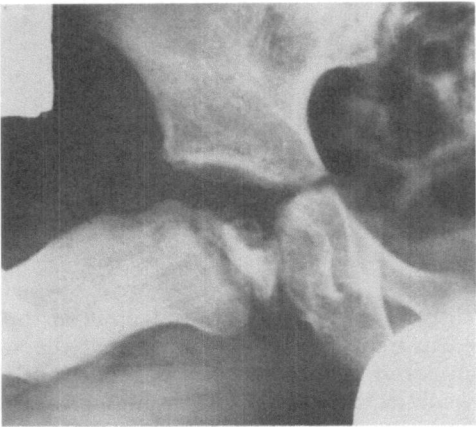

Fig. 8.1. A lateral view of the head of the femur showing that it is only the lateral part of the nucleus which is involved

between the lip of the acetabulum and the neck. The posteromedial vessels are much less vulnerable, and it is unusual for the posteromedial part of the nucleus to be involved in isolation. But in one-third of cases the whole of the nucleus is involved at the same time. It is difficult to see how such a thing could happen as a result of local trauma.

There is also great variation in the intensity of the ischaemia, so that in some the ischaemic changes will have cleared completely in 6–9 months (Figs. 8.2 and 8.3), whereas in others with apparently similar involvement the whole nucleus will ultimately be absorbed (Figs. 8.4 and 8.5). A possible explanation is that while the extent varies according to whether one or both leashes are involved, the intensity varies with the number of vessels involved in each leash. This would explain the great number of variants which are encountered in clinical experience.

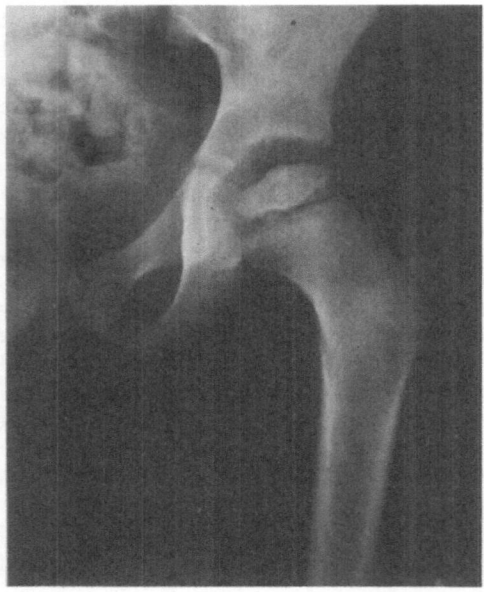

Fig. 8.2. Early but definite Perthes' changes seen in the hip of a girl aged 6 years

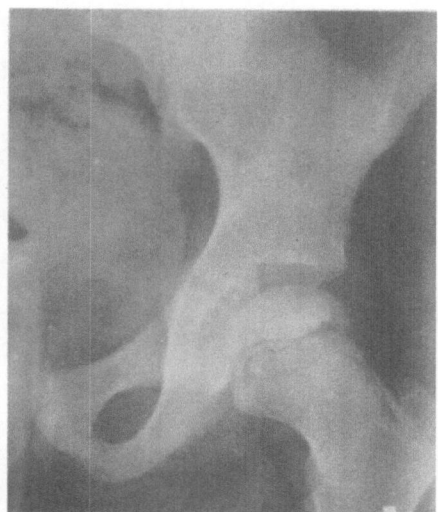

Fig. 8.3. Only 6 months later the condition shown in Fig. 8.2 has healed without treatment

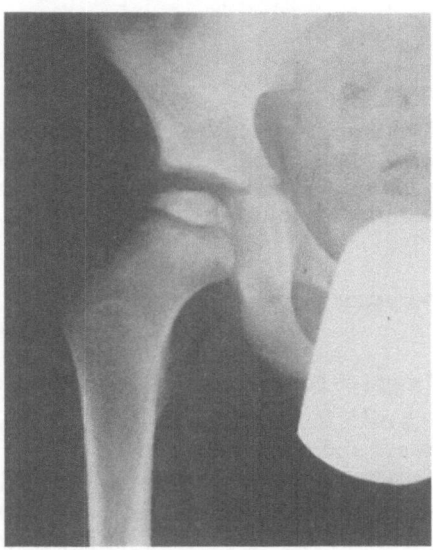

Fig. 8.4. Early Perthes' changes seen in the right hip of a boy aged 6 years

A further variant is introduced by involvement of the growth plate. There is little doubt that ischaemia of the nucleus will in some cases damage the growth plate (Glimcher 1977). This accounts for the broadening of the neck with shortening and, in the more extreme cases, premature fusion. These changes are well demonstrated in the case recorded by McKibbin and Ralis (1974). It is likely that the minor degree of deformity which persists after treatment in so many cases and which may take years to be completely remodelled is due to a minor degree of damage to the growth plate. It should not be overlooked that over-energetic and rough treatment can also damage the plate.

In radiographs taken early in the course of the disease it is usually impossible to distinguish between the different types. The most usual is that in which only the anterolateral part of the nucleus is affected, but it is very difficult to distinguish the

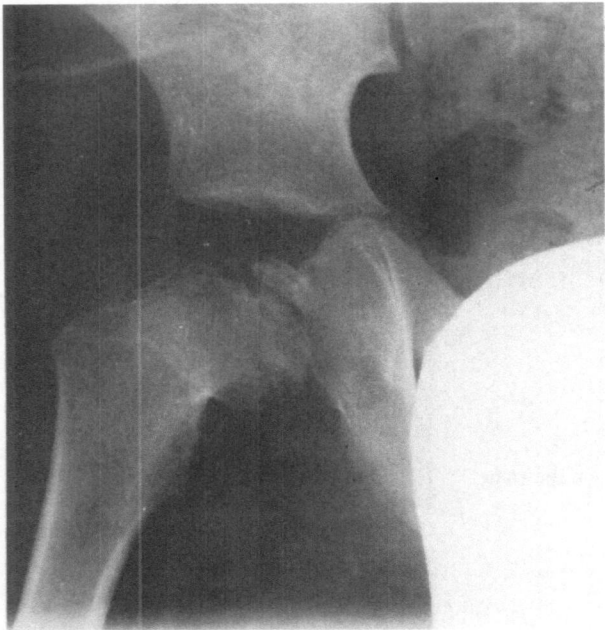

Fig. 8.5. The same case as in Fig. 8.4 after 15 months' treatment in broomstick plasters. The nucleus is almost absorbed

initial appearance from that seen in Fig. 8.4, which progressed to whole nucleus involvement (Fig. 8.5), or to distinguish either of them from that seen in Fig. 8.2, in which the lesion was transient and the ossific nucleus was restored to normal in 6 months without treatment (Fig. 8.3).

PATHOLOGY

Legg (1910) originally described the condition as passing through three phases.

1) The *ischaemic phase*, in which the ossific nucleus becomes radiologically slightly dense and almond-shaped.

2) The phase of *absorption*, in which the ischaemic bone is progressively absorbed, leaving behind variable amounts of viable bone depending on the intensity and extent of the ischaemia. This presents a mottled appearance often referred to mistakenly as fragmentation.

3) The phase of *re-ossification*, in which after absorption is complete new bone is laid down in many small nuclei presenting an appearance even more like fragmentation (Fig. 8.6) though it is in fact just the opposite. Re-ossification continues until consolidation is completed.

A fourth phase can now be added—the phase of *remodelling*. This phase continues far beyond the healing of the disease and beyond the cessation of growth (Somerville 1971).

These changes are seen more readily when the whole nucleus is involved than in where only a part is involved and where overlap will confuse the picture.

As already mentioned, in the early radiographs it is difficult to be certain of the extent or intensity of the ischaemia. Figure 8.4 shows the early changes in a boy aged 6 years who was treated with a short period of traction followed by a long period in broomstick plasters. The absorption of the nucleus was not complete for 15 months (Fig. 8.5). Three months later (Fig. 8.6) a radiograph showed that re-ossification had

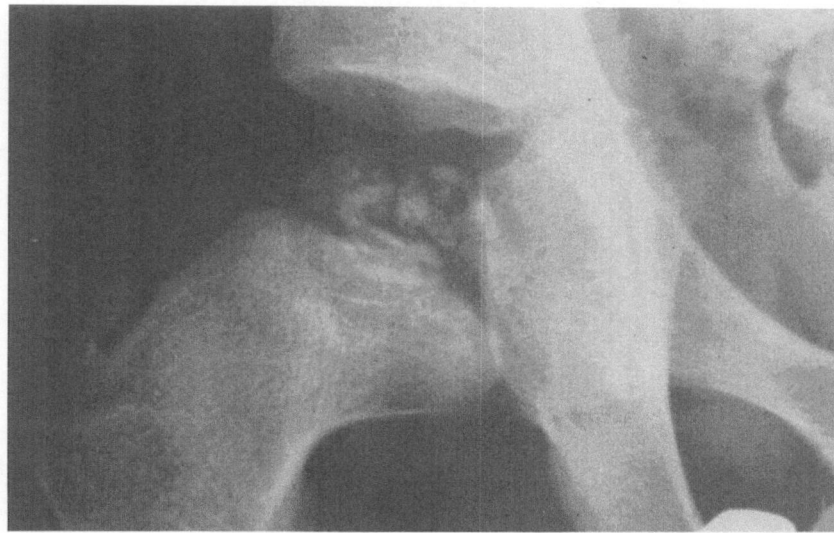

Fig. 8.6. Three months after the radiograph shown in Fig. 8.5 was taken the nucleus has reappeared in the form of multiple small centres of ossification

started in the form of multiple ossific nuclei in the shape of a normal nucleus. Eight months later these nuclei were seen to be fusing together, and at the age of 16 years consolidation was complete (Fig. 8.7), but the shape of the head was not normal, being too broad and a little shallow. Four years later, at the age of 20, further remodelling had taken place and the hip was indistinguishable from normal when compared with the opposite side (Fig. 8.8). When only a part of the nucleus is involved the sequence is probably the same but the appearance is confused by the overlap of the normal parts of the nucleus.

This sequence raises certain interesting points:

1) When the new ossific nucleus appeared it was not only the shape of the previous one but had also grown to the size it would have been after a period of 18 months if no ischaemia had ever occurred. This can only mean that the femoral head has been alive and quite unaffected by the changes in the ossific nucleus and the cartilage elements have gone on growing at the normal rate. This accounts for the apparent widening of the joint space seen in early radiographs.

2) Perthes' disease must not be confused with avascular necrosis of the femoral head. Avascular necrosis involves death of the femoral head, whereas in Perthes' disease the ischaemia involves the ossific nucleus only, the rest of the head—the cartilaginous part—being unaffected, so that in Perthes' disease reossification will always take place; if it does not then the condition is not Perthes' disease but avascular necrosis.

3) The ischaemia must be of short duration because the circulation must be restored before the absorption can begin.

4) What replaces the absorbed bone? Presumably fibrous tissue. If it is fibrous tissue it will not grow and it would be most unlikely that new bone would grow in it.

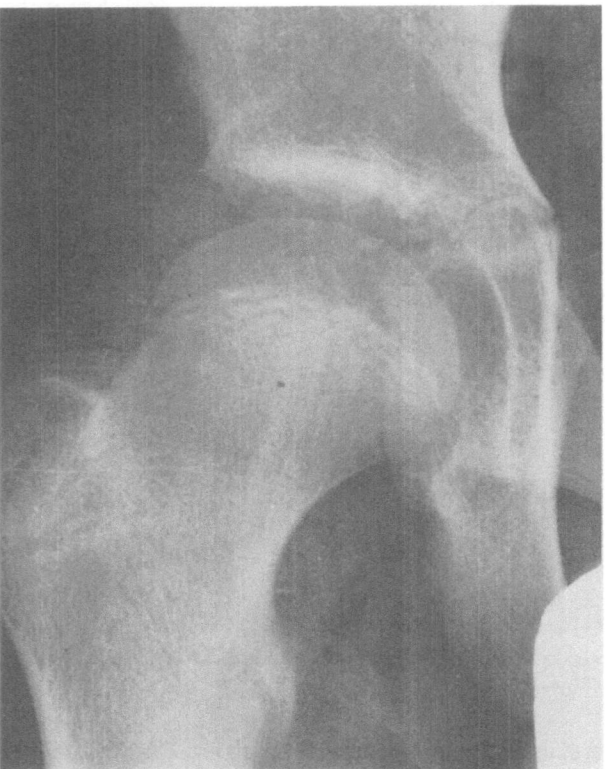

Fig. 8.7. At the age of 16 years the nucleus is well consolidated but the head is broad and the nucleus shallow in the hip shown in Figs. 8.6 and 8.7

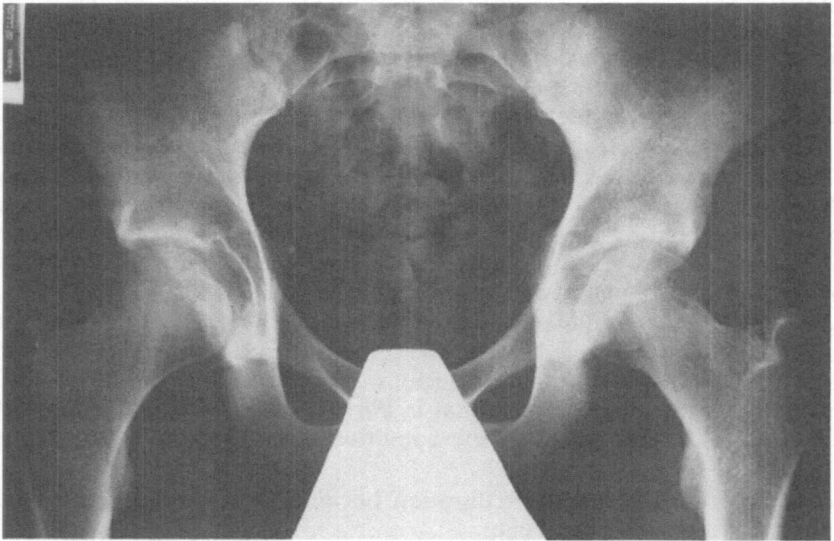

Fig. 8.8. Four years after the radiograph shown in Fig. 8.7 was taken the head and neck are indistinguishable from normal

5) The new bone must be laid down in the bone-bearing cartilaginous layer around the ischaemic nucleus which has continued growing normally.

6) The sequence of events suggests that re-ossification does not start until absorption is completed. It does not seem possible that blood vessels and cells which were concerned with absorption up to a certain time can suddenly change their characteristics and start laying down new bone. It is more likely that this observation is coincidental. It is only by the time absorption is complete that sufficient bone-forming cartilage has developed in which the multiple ossific nuclei can be laid down.

7) This layer of cartilage will be in the form of a dome with the old fibrous tissue in the middle. Subsequent development suggests that bone gradually invades the fibrous tissue, which ultimately disappears though its outline may persist for a while as the 'head within a head' mentioned by Salter (1966).

8) The presence of some deformity of the head and neck persisting after consolidation is complete, which is not uncommon, is an indication of some damage to the growth plate, however slight.

9) The remodelling of the head long after consolidation is complete and well beyond the cessation of growth can only be achieved in the presence of normal joint mechanics. Without this deterioration must occur.

The sequence of events as described is shown diagrammatically in Fig. 8.9.

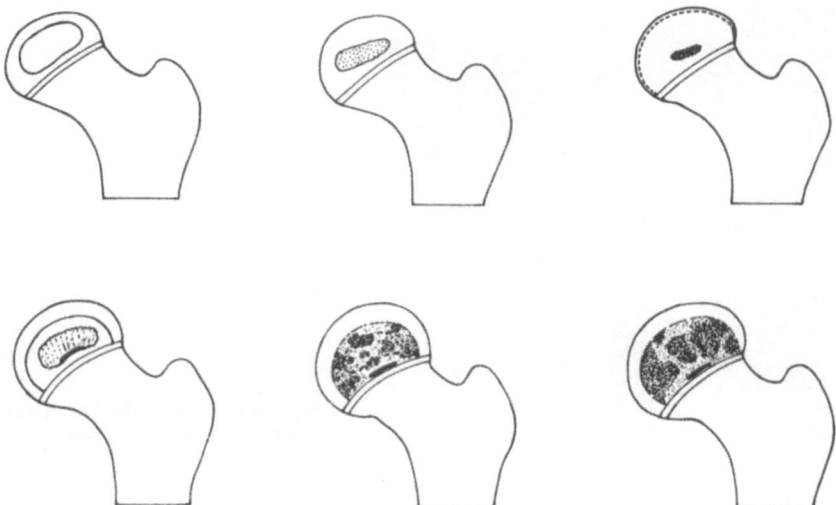

Fig. 8.9. The sequence of events in this severe case, shown diagrammatically, is probably similar to the changes seen in almost all cases of Perthes' disease, but the course is often much modified by the extent and severity of the condition

Subluxation

It is only during the last few years that the importance of subluxation has been fully appreciated. The cause for it is by no means clear, though it is possible that the same process as caused the ischaemia also caused some softening of the capsule, rendering it temporarily more stretchable than normal, and once it has stretched it remains stretched. There is no evidence to suggest that the subluxation precedes the ischaemia; if this were so there would be some stigma to indicate it. The incidence of

Perthes' disease developing in a previously subluxated hip must be extremely rare. In the present series there were seven hips with well-marked ischaemic changes in which there was no evidence of subluxation and in which no treatment was necessary, and there were a further three hips in which there was at first no evidence of subluxation but in which it developed later, so that treatment became necessary. Boldero and Kemp (1966) showed that some degree of displacement could appear before the ischaemia became radiologically apparent; indeed they suggested that the presence of this very slight displacement was an indication that ischaemia might become apparent later.

The degree of subluxation is rarely more than minimal and sometimes it may be missed unless it is carefully looked for. Radiologically the head may be seen extending a little further laterally beyond the lip of the acetabulum than on the other side, but the increased gap between the head and the dew-drop in the medial wall of the acetabulum is more obvious (Fig. 8.10). The appearance suggests that the head is

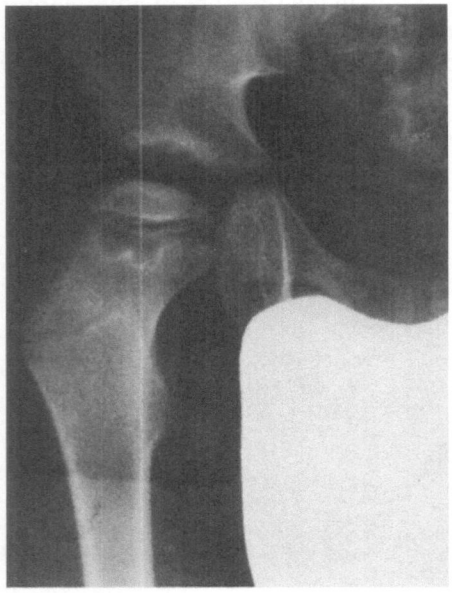

Fig. 8.10. Early Perthes' changes seen in the hip of a boy aged 6 years. The degree of subluxation is clear

extruded laterally by some radiolucent space occupying tissue sometimes thought to be a hypertrophied fat pad or synovium. But the appearance is probably misleading. It is more likely that the displacement is similar to the minor degree of displacement seen in congenital subluxation, in which the apparent lateral displacement is the result of lateral rotation. Such a view is supported by two observations. Firstly, very often the only physical sign in Perthes' disease is loss of medial rotation. This is even more constant than is the loss of some degree of abduction and is likely to be evidence of anterior displacement, so that the degree of displacement may be rather greater than the radiograph suggests. And, secondly, such displacement is more readily reduced by simple medial rotation than by abduction alone, but as will be shown, is reduced best of all by a combination of the two (Fig. 8.11).

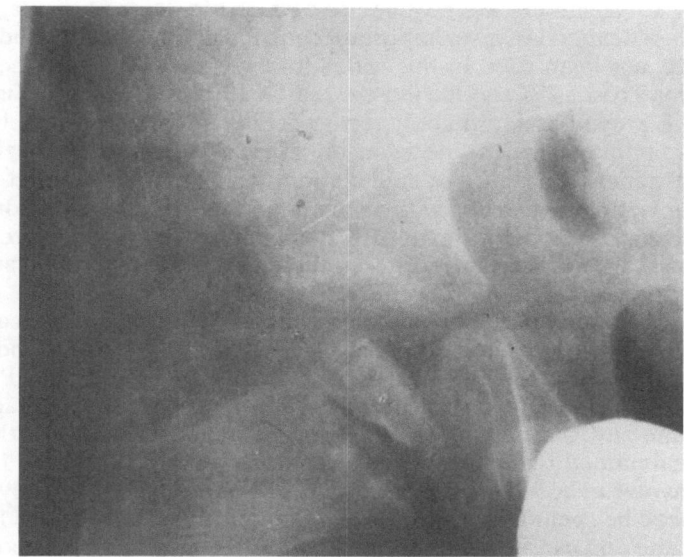

Fig. 8.11. The same hip as shown in Fig. 8.10, the leg in plaster with the hip medially rotated and slightly abducted. The subluxation has been reduced

TREATMENT

Since the initial description of the condition by Legg (1910), treatment has always been based on the principle that relief of pressure on the femoral head should be ensured while it was soft, until re-ossification had reached a point when it was once more safe to allow weight-bearing, even though this might take several years. The methods used varied from simple recumbency or recumbency with traction, either straight or in abduction, to non-weight-bearing appliances such as pattern-ended calipers or Snyder's slings.

A comparison carried out by Lauritzen (1975) showed little difference between the methods, but there was a preference for those which involved recumbency over those involving calipers and slings.

In the 1920s A. O. Parker, working in Cardiff and Oswestry, introduced the use of broomstick plasters (Fig. 5.35) to maintain the hips in full medial rotation and abduction with the object of providing the maximum coverage of the femoral head and at the same time allowing movement which would encourage active moulding of the softened head while re-ossification was taking place. This procedure had the added advantage that it reduced the subluxation, and although it took a long time it produced excellent results. A similar procedure, which allowed the patient some degree of ambulation, was described by Petrie and Bitenc (1971).

Evans and Lloyd-Roberts (1958) pointed out that there were many patients with Perthes' hips which did not need to be treated, who did very well if left alone to lead a normal life. Since then the great question has been whether to treat or not to treat.

In an attempt to resolve this problem Catterall (1971), after an extensive survey of hips treated at The Hospital for Sick Children, Great Ormond Street and elsewhere, evolved a classification based on the severity and type of ischaemia. He was able to divide them into four groups from which an assessment could be made as to whether or not treatment was required and which hips were particularly at risk. Although the classification is a most important contribution to our knowledge of Perthes' disease it has not been used in this series for two reasons. Firstly because the first hip was treated in 1957 and the most recent in 1973, and secondly because the classification has proved easier to apply retrospectively than prospectively.

In this series the decision on whether to treat has been based purely on the presence or absence of subluxation. It was considered that if the eccentric type of movement associated with even minor degrees of subluxation could, in an otherwise normal joint, cause extensive deformity it was even more likely to do so in the presence of ischaemia. It was thought that if the subluxation was corrected the deformity might be prevented.

The reduction of subluxation seldom presents any difficulty. It can be achieved quite easily by simple medial rotation with or without abduction (Figs. 8.10 and 8.11). The problem is how to maintain the reduction. Parker and later Petrie demonstrated how this could be done with external splintage but this takes a long time and can disrupt a young patient's childhood. Reduction can be equally well maintained by means of a high femoral osteotomy (Axer 1965, 1973), which will involve a short period of treatment, i.e., about 10 weeks; only a small part of this time need be spent in hospital, after which the child can resume his normal activity. The same end can be achieved by means of an innominate osteotomy (Salter 1966).

In this series a high femoral osteotomy has been used throughout because we have found it simpler and more reliable, though it should be mentioned that if more than 25° or 30° of varus is necessary to obtain adequate coverage then it will be wise to combine femoral osteotomy with a pelvic osteotomy. This is rarely necessary and was not done in the series described.

TECHNIQUE

At the time of admission to hospital the child is allowed to settle down for a few days, after which simple skin traction is applied to the leg until spasm has been relieved. This is followed by traction in increasing abduction, in this series on a frame. Abduction is gradually increased until there is at least 100° between the legs, though with care to ensure that at no time is any force used.

Under anaesthesia the child is removed from the frame and put into a plaster spica with the hips in 45° of abduction and as much medial rotation as can be obtained without using force. This is repeated 2 weeks later, when it will be possible to obtain about 45° of medial rotation without using force. Two weeks later the plaster is removed. Broomstick plasters can be used just as well as a spica.

Initially it was customary to take radiographs in medial rotation with and without abduction to determine whether the osteotomy should be rotation only or rotation with varus. When it became apparent that the results of rotation with varus were so much better than the results of rotation only this was discontinued.

The technique of osteotomy is the same as that described for congenital dislocation of the hip, but in Perthes' disease there is no deformity to be corrected, so that the rotation must be limited to no more than 30° and the varus to 20°, except in exceptional circumstances. In Perthes' disease an excessive degree of varus will not correct as it usually will in congenital dislocation of the hip. This is probably because the patients are in an older age group and because in many cases of Perthes' disease there is some interference with the growth plate; not sufficient to prevent normal growth but enough to prevent overgrowth. The use of the trochanteric flare to provide 15°–20° of varus without bending the plate (p. 58 and Figs. 4.22 and 4.23) is particularly useful in Perthes' disease.

At 6–8 weeks after operation, depending on the age of the child, when the osteotomy is united, the plaster is removed and the child is allowed to mobilise and resume full normal activity as soon as possible without any restrictions or splintage, regardless of the radiological appearance.

FOLLOW-UP

Forty-five hips treated in this way have been followed up for a maximum of 20 years and a minimum of 4 years (Somerville 1980). This follow-up has shown that the osteotomy has little if any effect on the rate of re-ossification, so that the hip will still pass through all the stages previously described before re-ossification and re-modelling take place.

Fig. 8.12 shows the hip of a child aged 6 years with early Perthes' changes for which an osteotomy was performed because of the minor degree of subluxation which was present. One year later about 50% of the nucleus had been absorbed (Fig. 8.13). Subsequent radiographs at yearly intervals show re-ossification progressively taking place (Fig. 8.14), but it was not until 5 years after osteotomy that consolidation was complete (Fig. 8.15); however, the head was still broad and the epiphysis shallow. During the next 6 years gradual remodelling has taken place so that by the age of 17 the hip is normal (Fig. 8.16). This hip has followed the course of many which have progressed in a straightforward manner.

It is commonly believed that there are a number of factors which have an effect on the prognosis for better or for worse.

Factors Affecting the Prognosis

AGE

The age at which the diagnosis is made is frequently confused with the age at which

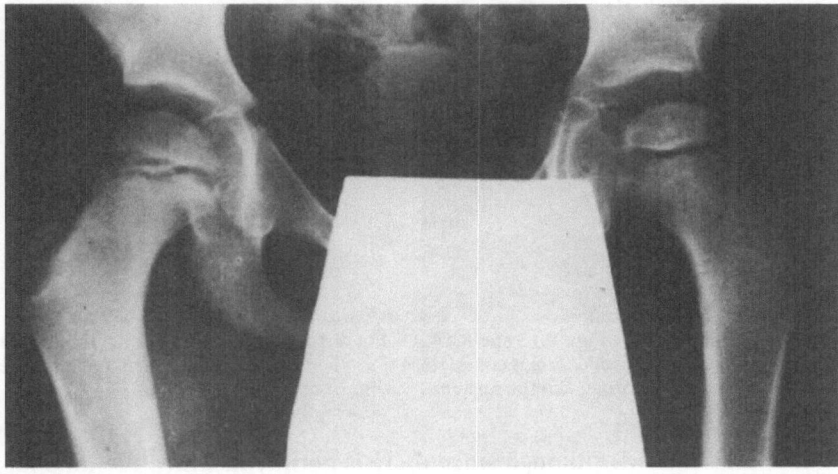

Fig. 8.12. Early Perthes' disease in the left hip with a minor degree of subluxation, which is very obvious on comparison with the normal hip

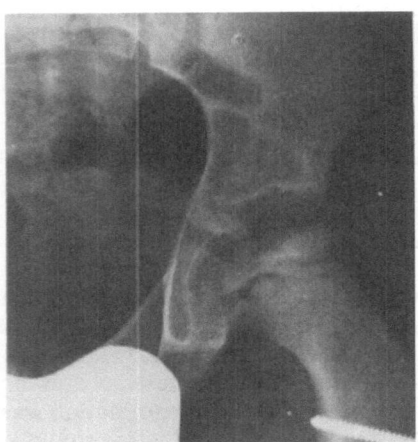

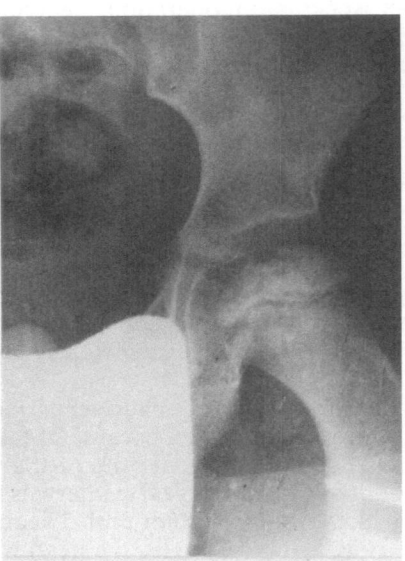

Fig. 8.13. One year after osteotomy performed to correct the deformity shown in Fig. 8.12, about half the nucleus has been absorbed

Fig. 8.14. Sixteen months after the radiograph shown in Fig. 8.13 was taken the defect is seen to be filling in from the periphery

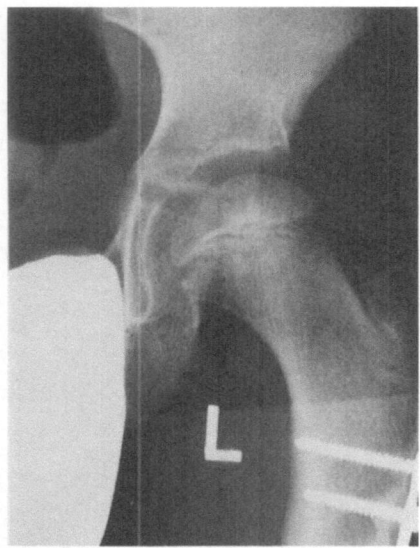

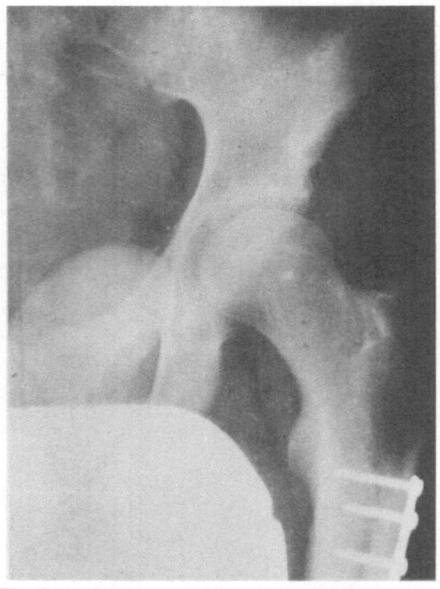

Fig. 8.15. Same hip as in Figs. 8.13 and 8.14. Two years later the consolidation is complete but the head is a little broad and the nucleus a little shallow

Fig. 8.16. Seven years after the radiograph shown in Fig. 8.15 was taken, the left hip is almost normal at the age of 17

the disease started, although since there is no way in which the time lapse between onset and diagnosis can be estimated all that can be done is to estimate the effect of age at the time of treatment. In this series, as can be seen in Table 8.1, the age at the

Table 8.1. The effect of age on the result of treatment for Perthes' disease

	Results		
	Good	Fair	Poor
Treated hips	33	7	5
Total 45			
Average age	6.5	7.5	6.5
Untreated hips	6	0	1
Total 7			
Average age 7			

time of treatment has had comparatively little effect on the result. A case of Perthes' disease diagnosed at the age of 8 years and with the changes already far advanced (Figs. 8.17 and 8.18) made an excellent recovery over a period of 8 years (Fig. 8.19). Even in a boy aged 11 years with very severe changes (Fig. 8.20) and true deformity of the femoral head, as seen in an arthrogram (Fig. 8.21), a remarkable improvement took place over a period of 6 years, although the result has been marred by damaged to the growth plate (Fig. 8.22). At the lower end of the scale a child diagnosed at the age of 4 with only moderate changes then present had a disappointing result after exactly the same treatment.

EXTENT OF INVOLVEMENT

In this series there is little to suggest that total involvement of the nucleus indicates results different from those in which involvement has been only partial. A boy of 8 years of age was found at diagnosis to have total nucleus involvement (Fig. 8.23). After a rotation osteotomy with varus the head was well contained although the

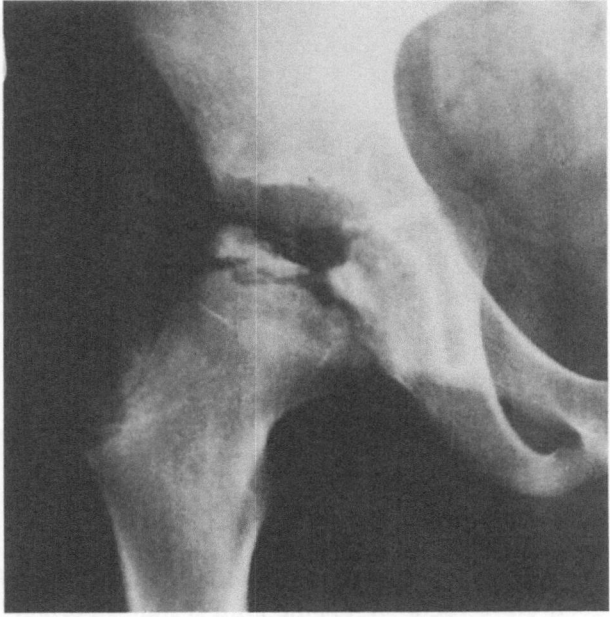

Fig. 8.17. Advanced Perthes' changes in the right hip of a boy aged 8 years

damage to the nucleus was very severe (Fig. 8.24). Twenty years after the osteotomy the hip was congruous although the neck was a little short and the head a little broad due to mild damage to the growth plate (Fig. 8.25). The appearance suggests that the acetabulum is slightly deformed, but the other acetabulum is just the same shape. This patient was a professional footballer for 10 years.

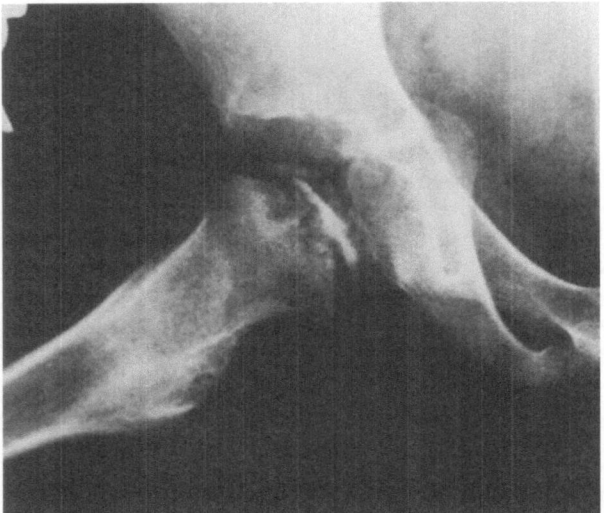

Fig. 8.18. The lateral view of the same hip as illustrated in Fig. 8.17 shows the extent of the damage

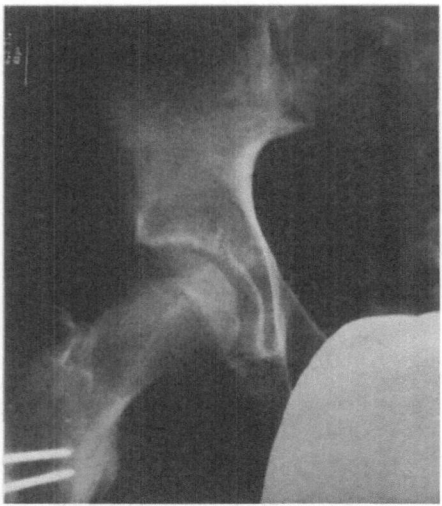

Fig. 8.19. Eight years after treatment the hip shown in Figs. 8.17 and 8.18 is restored to normal

A younger child aged 4½ years already had extensive changes when first seen, with whole nucleus involvement (Fig. 8.26). This boy also had considerable pain in the hip. Sixteen months after osteotomy there was great improvement (Fig. 8.27) and 11 years after treatment the hip joint is almost normal (Fig. 8.28). There is still a small increase in the varus although this is improving.

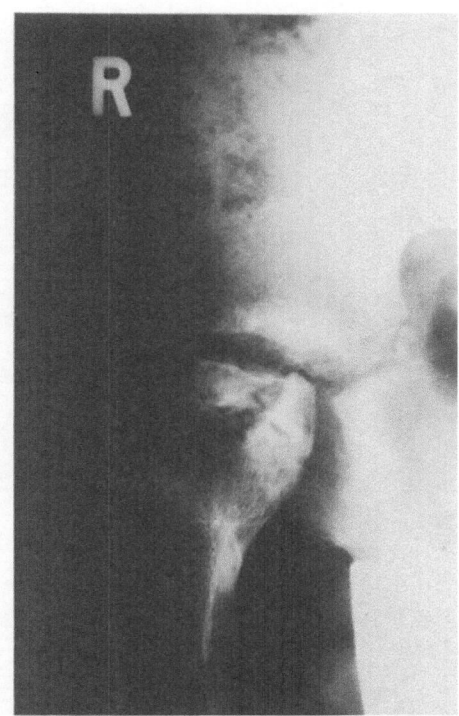

Fig. 8.20. Very severe changes seen in the right hip of a boy aged 11 years

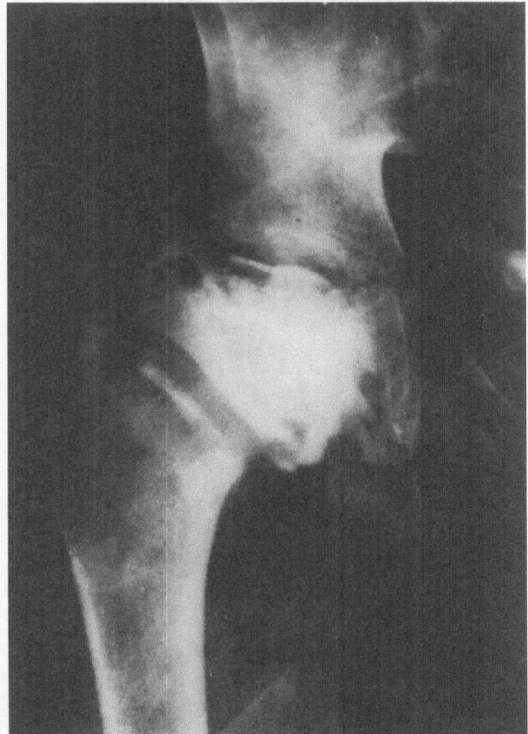

Fig. 8.21. An arthrogram of the hip illustrated in Fig. 8.20 shows that there is marked deformity of the head

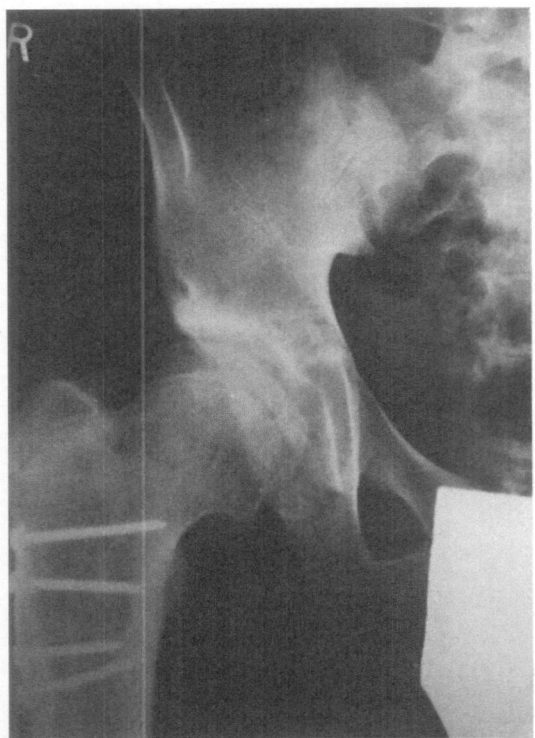

Fig. 8.22. Six years after the osteotomy, although there has obviously been much damage to the growth plate, resulting in shortness of the neck, which is also broad, the head is round and congruous with the acetabulum

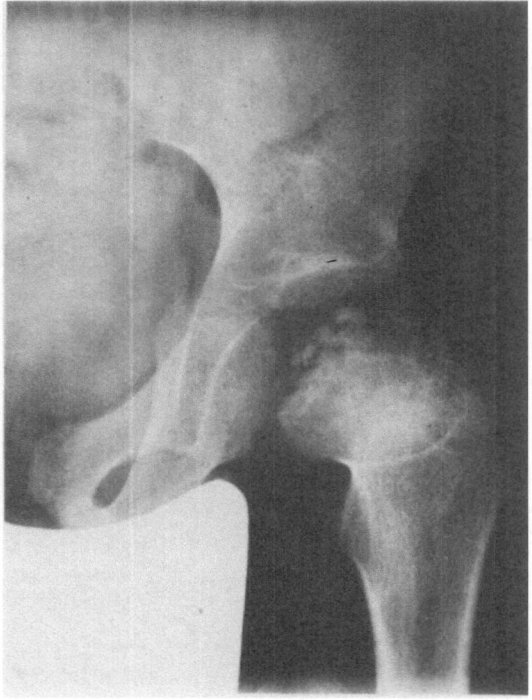

Fig. 8.23. The hip of a boy aged 8 years with severe changes well advanced and with marked subluxation

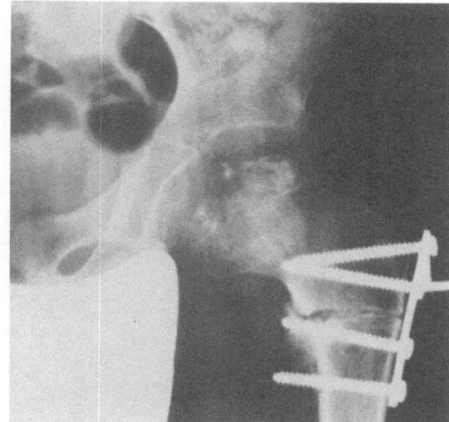

Fig. 8.24. The same hip as in Fig. 8.23, shortly after rotation and varus osteotomy. The varus has been achieved with a straight plate by making use of the flare of the trochanter ▶

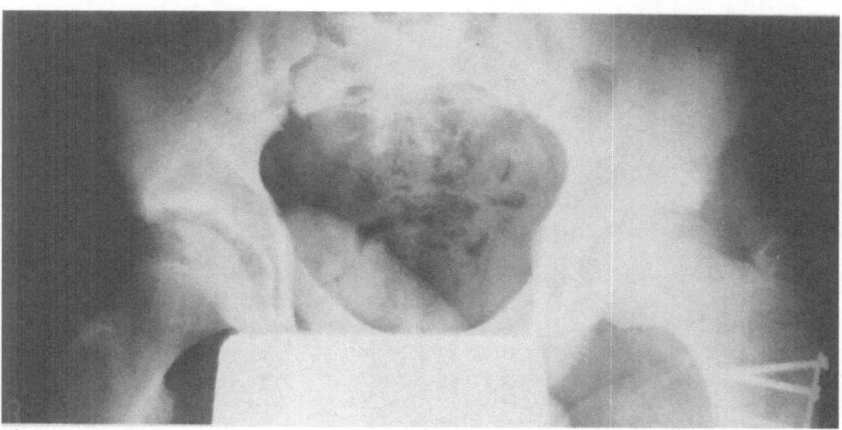

Fig. 8.25. Twenty years after osteotomy on the hip shown in Fig. 8.24 there is only a minor degree of stigma due to very minor involvement of the growth plate

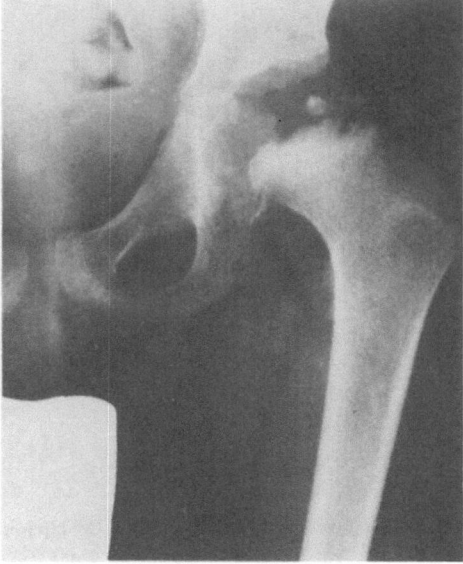

Fig. 8.26. Very severe changes in the left hip of a boy at the age of 4

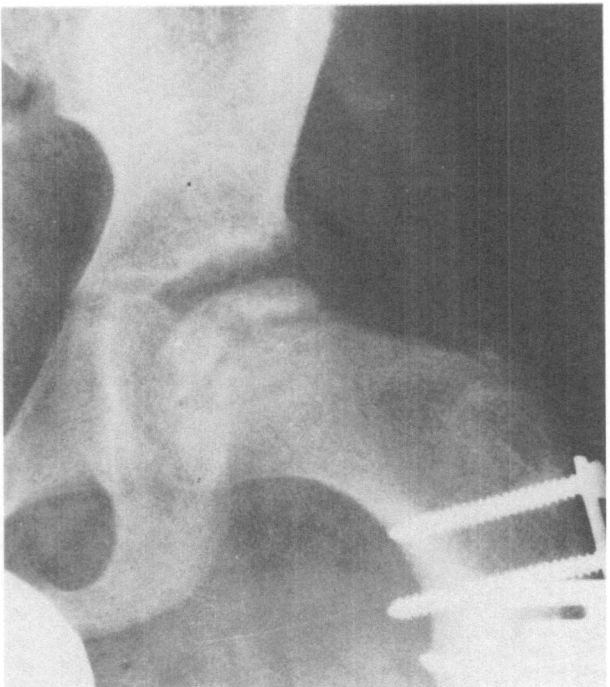

Fig. 8.27. The same case as in Fig. 8.26, seen 16 months after osteotomy and showing great improvement

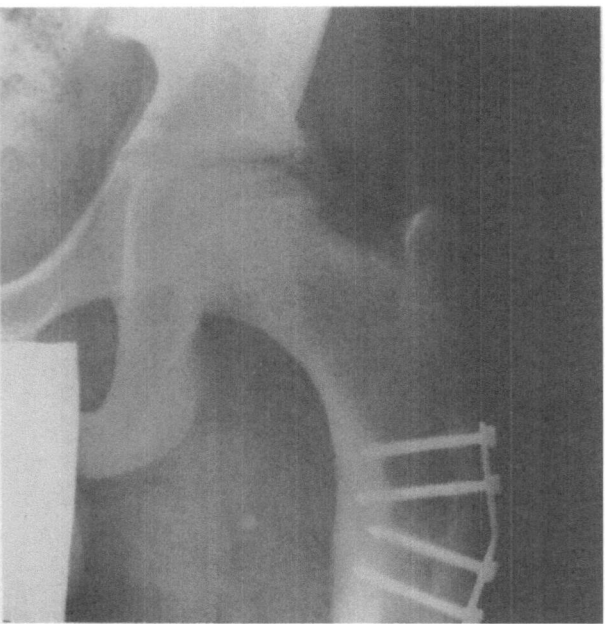

Fig. 8.28. Eleven years after treatment the hip joint seen in Figs. 8.26 and 8.27 is almost normal although there is still some excess varus

PHASE OF THE LESION AT DIAGNOSIS

In the belief that deformity was due to the direct effect of pressure, early diagnosis and treatment have always been considered essential to reduce it to the minimum. Results obtained in this series strongly suggest that although early treatment is no doubt desirable it is not as important as had been supposed. Table 8.2 shows that

Table 8.2. The effect of the phase of Perthes' disease at diagnosis on the result of treatment

Phase at diagnosis	Results		
	Good	Fair	Poor
Advanced	12 (66.3%)	3 (16.5%)	3 (16.5%)
Moderate	12 (80%)	2 (13.5%)	1 (6.5%)
Early	9 (75%)	2 (16.5%)	1 (8.5%)
Total	33	7	5

although the results in those treated when the lesion was already advanced are not quite as good as those treated when the lesion was only moderately advanced or early, the difference is much less marked than might have been expected. Three hips not included in this series had reached the phase of consolidation with marked deformity before the diagnosis was made: osteotomy was not beneficial and is probably contraindicated in this phase.

OSTEOTOMY

It is very difficult to obtain clear evidence of the effect of osteotomy on the rate of recovery, because there is such a wide variation from one case to another. In this series there is no evidence to show that osteotomy has any effect on the rate of recovery. A boy aged 5 years had moderate involvement (Fig. 8.29). Two years later there was only very minor improvement (Fig. 8.30). It took a further 5 years

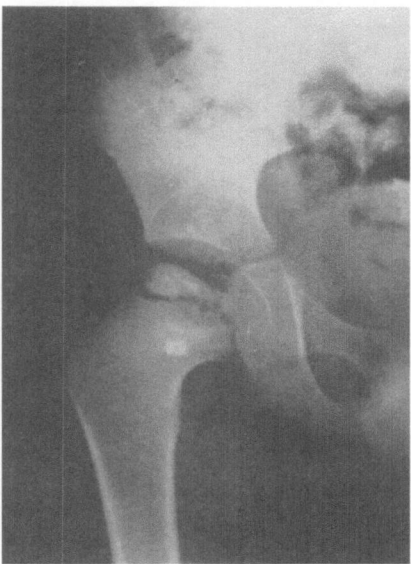

Fig. 8.29. Perthes' changes involving the whole of the nucleus in a boy aged 5 years

before consolidation was complete, but the result at 12 years was satisfactory (Fig. 8.31). Another boy, aged 10 years, had well-advanced changes at the time of diagnosis (Fig. 8.32) and only 6 months after the osteotomy consolidation was seen to be well advanced (Fig. 8.33). In another case widespread changes were seen in the ossific nucleus of a girl aged 4 (Fig. 8.34). Only 2 months after osteotomy the appearance in the radiograph suggested that revascularisation was well advanced (Fig. 8.35). The hip continued to develop normally without ever passing through the usual phases (Fig. 8.36). In the great majority of cases from diagnosis and osteotomy to consolidation has taken about 3 years, with remodelling continuing for many

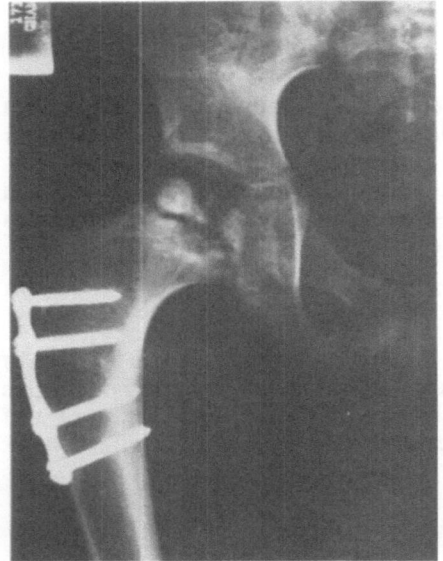

Fig. 8.30. Two years after the osteotomy on the hip shown in Fig. 8.29 there is surprisingly little improvement

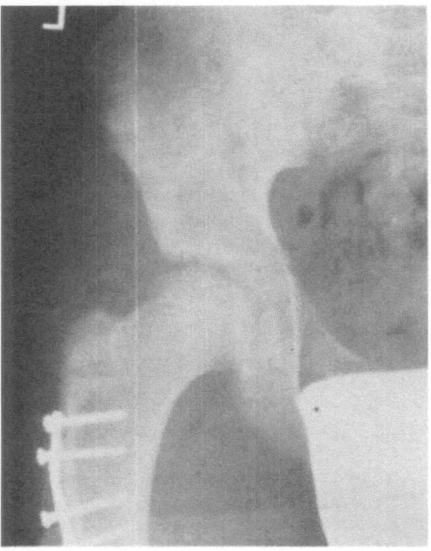

Fig. 8.31. A further 6 years after the radiograph shown in Fig. 8.30 was taken the head and acetabulum are well developed

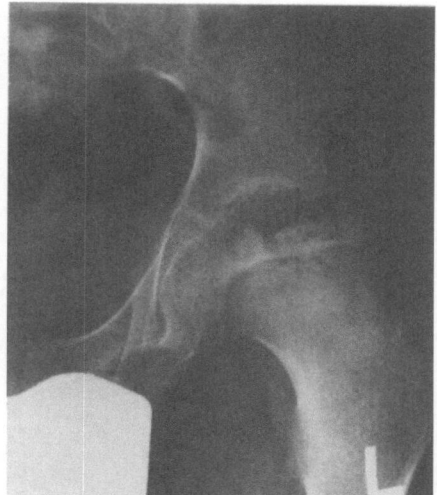

Fig. 8.32. Advanced changes are seen in the head of the left hip of a boy aged 10 years. The appearance suggests collapse

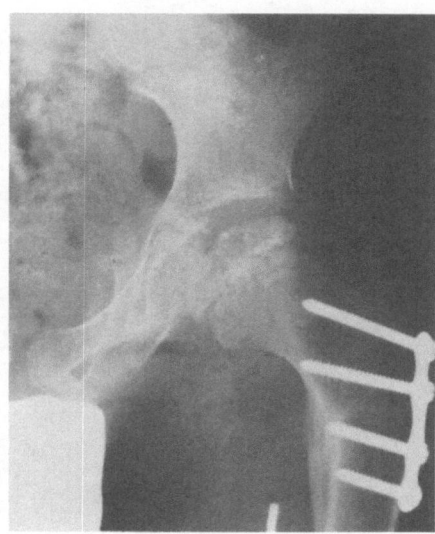

Fig. 8.33. The same hip as in Fig. 8.32 only 6 months after the radiograph in Fig. 8.32 was taken, showing extensive re-ossification. If there was any collapse it must have been minimal. The appearance in the previous radiograph must have been due to absorption

years afterwards. This is very comparable to the time required in hips treated by bloodless methods.

SEVERITY OF SYMPTOMS

In the great majority of cases symptoms at the time of diagnosis were minimal, and in some nonexistent. In a few cases, however, symptoms were severe. The hip of the boy shown in Fig. 8.25 was very painful and the range of movement was restricted by spasm. The result (Fig. 8.27) was excellent. In another child, aged 11 years (Figs. 8.37 and 8.38), the hip was very painful and there was very little movement because of severe spasm. Seven years after osteotomy (Fig. 8.39) a good congruous hip has developed although the head is still a little big and the neck slightly short due to minor damage to the growth plate. A full range of movement has been restored.

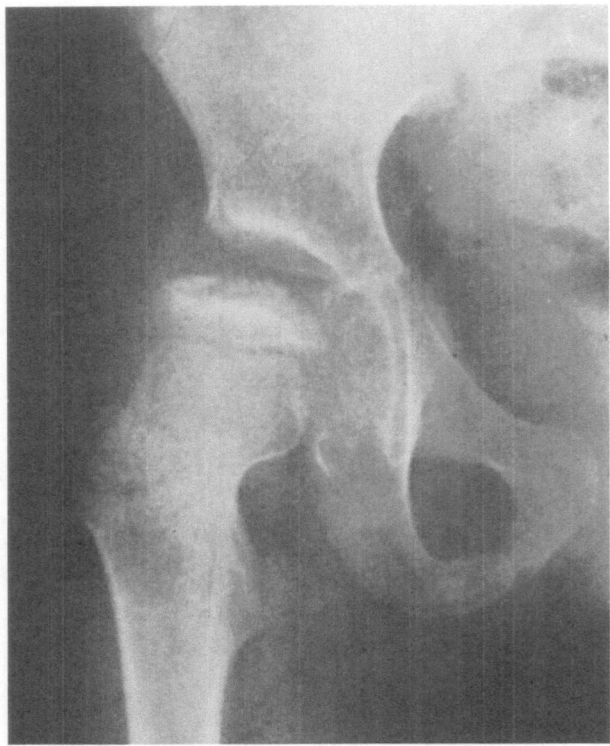

Fig. 8.34. Obvious changes in the right hip of a girl aged 4

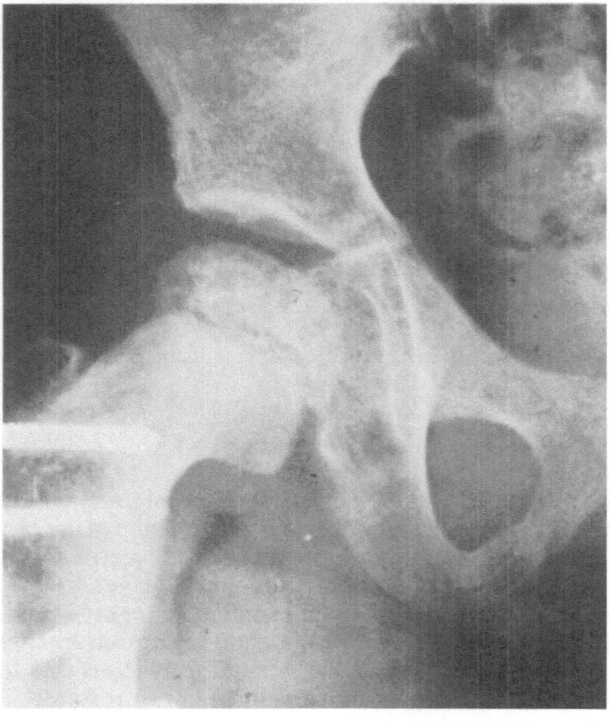

Fig. 8.35. Two months after the radiograph in Fig. 8.34 was taken the ossification is well advanced

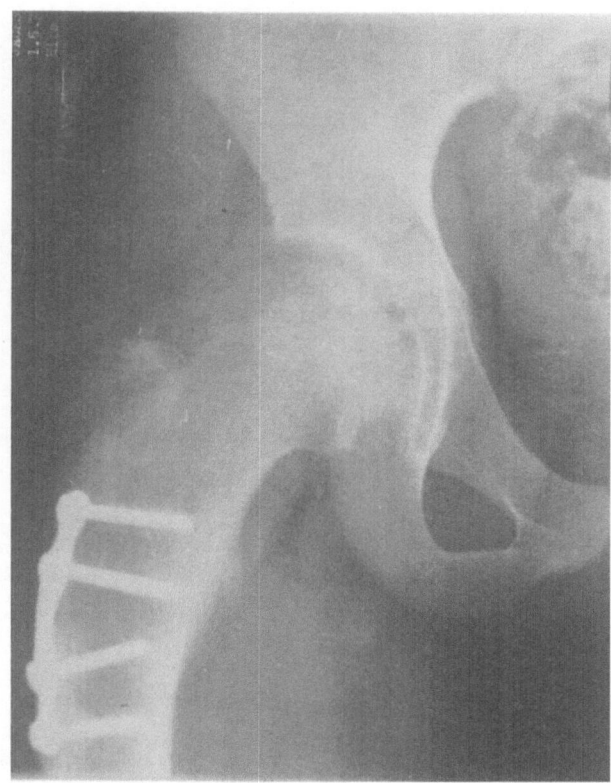

Fig. 8.36. Many years later the hip seen in Figs. 8.34 and 8.35 is normal

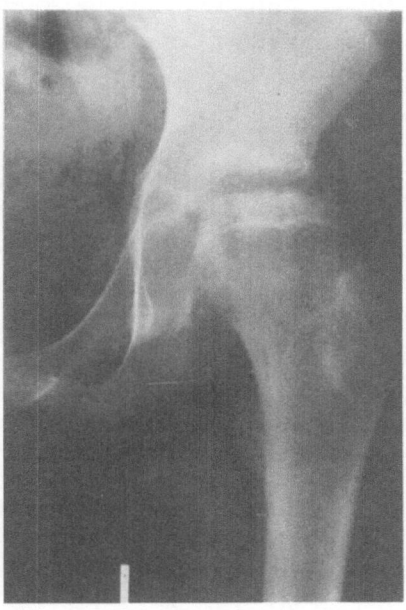

Fig. 8.37. Extensive changes in the nucleus
apparently involving the metaphysis. The hip was
very painful

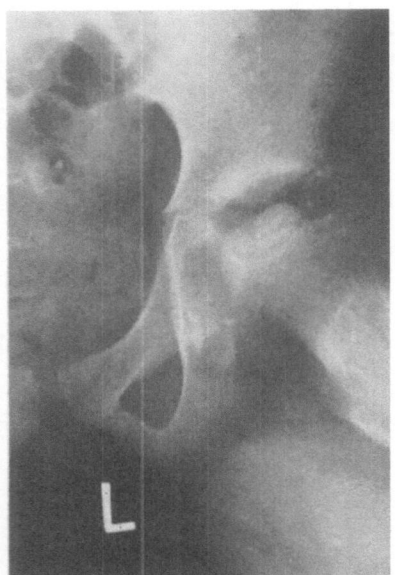

Fig. 8.38. The lateral view shows the extent of the lesion seen in Fig. 8.37 more clearly

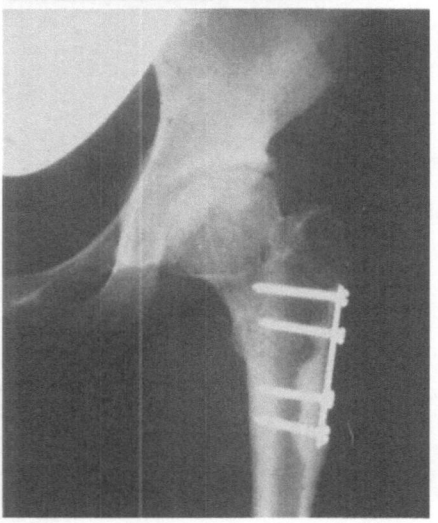

Fig. 8.39. The same hip as seen in Figs. 8.37 and 8.38 seven years later. There has been great improvement but the result is marred by premature fusion of the epiphyseal plate

WHAT DOES HAVE AN EFFECT ON THE RESULT?

Since so many factors seem to have surprisingly little effect on the result it is necessary to consider what factors will influence it. It seems likely that there are two: subluxation and damage to the growth plate.

Subluxation is the more common. This is fortunate because while nothing can be done to help damage to the growth plate, subluxation can be corrected, as has been explained, and in the majority of cases this will lead to a satisfactory result even in the most unlikely cases. In hips in which there is no subluxation no treatment is required and the child may be allowed to continue to lead a normal active life without

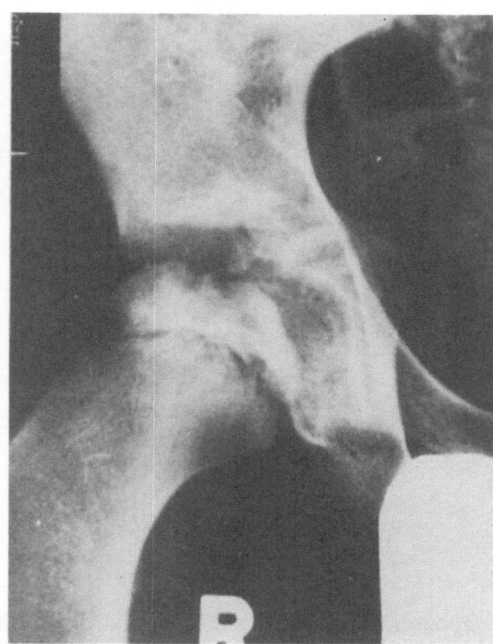

Fig. 8.40. Perthes' changes but without subluxation

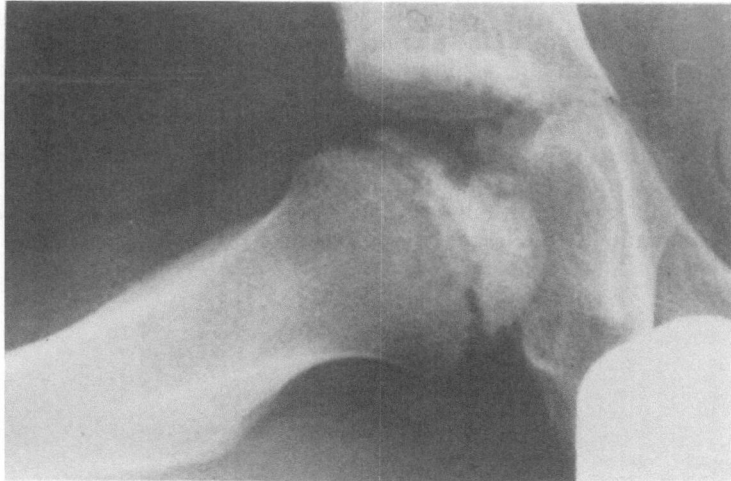

Fig. 8.41. The lateral view of the hip shown in Fig. 8.40 shows that only half the nucleus is involved

restraint, but the hip must be watched carefully because subluxation may develop later, and if it does osteotomy will become necessary to correct it. Figures 8.40 and 8.41 show the hip of a child with well-marked ischaemic changes but no evidence of subluxation, and there was a full range of movement including medial rotation. Such a hip requires no treatment and in this case the result was excellent (Fig. 8.42). It seems possible that the different categories described by Catterall (1971) as relevant to the prognosis following ischaemic changes are simply an indication that subluxation is more likely to occur in grades 3 and 4 and less likely in grades 1 and 2. But it is

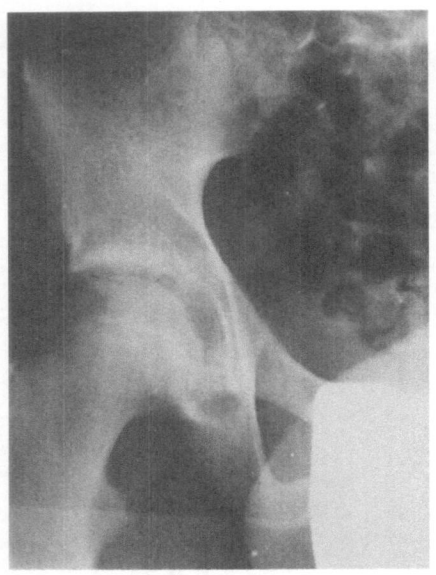

Fig. 8.42. Complete healing has taken place without treatment in the hip shown in Figs. 8.40 and 8.41

our experience that it is the subluxation which really matters rather than the severity of the ischaemia.

While it is easy to diagnose subluxation, it is extremely difficult to diagnose, in advance, damage to the growth plate, and it is damage to the growth plate which, being irreversible, is so important. It seems to occur to a major degree in about 10% of cases and in a lesser degree in a further 10%.

The initial radiograph of the hip of one child (Fig. 8.43) showed severe involvement of the ossific nucleus with subluxation, and the changes appeared to extend into the neck with involvement of the growth plate. But 8 years later (Fig. 8.44) the hip had developed normally with no suggestion of shortening of the femoral neck or broadening of the head. In another case the radiograph suggested sclerosis of the

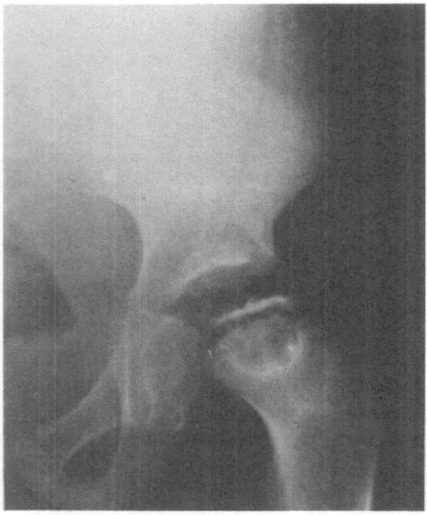

Fig. 8.43. Extensive and advanced changes in the left hip of a girl. The appearances suggest that the metaphysis may be involved

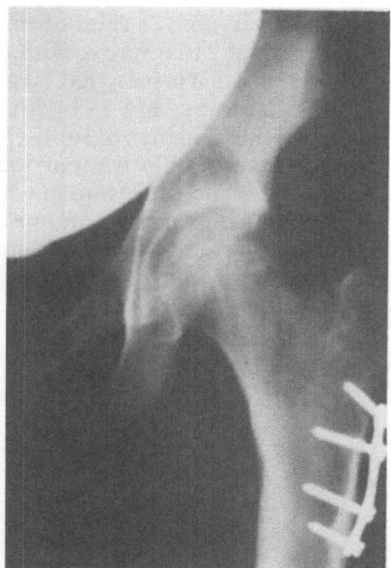

Fig. 8.44. The radiograph 8 years after that seen in Fig. 8.43 shows complete healing with no suggestion of damage to the growth plate

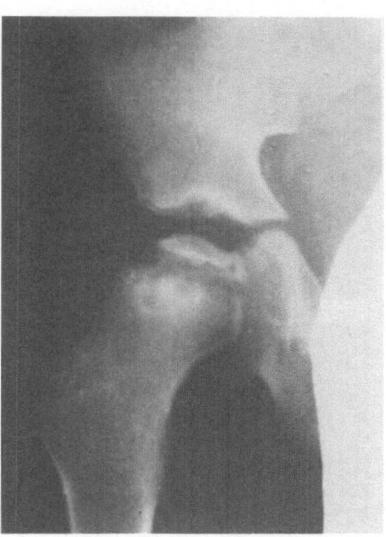

Fig. 8.45. Similar changes to those seen in the case illustrated in Figs. 8.43 and 8.44, but not quite so severe, in a boy aged 7

metaphysis (Fig. 8.45), which could indicate damage to the plate. Six months later (Fig. 8.46) the appearance suggested that the result must surely be a failure, but by 6 years later (Fig. 8.47) there was a great improvement, although the epiphysis was narrow and the head broad. There must have been some damage to the plate but recovery is still taking place. Very similar changes were seen in the hip of a boy aged 8 (Fig. 8.48), but 3 years later it was obvious that considerable damage had been done to the growth plate, resulting in growth deformity of the head and shortening of the neck; the head was only partially covered (Fig. 8.49). Six years later, with continuous use the whole joint had greatly improved (Fig. 8.50). The head was more circular and was better covered by the acetabular roof, although the neck remained short. There can be little doubt that there has been severe damage to the growth plate producing the deformity, but in spite of this the correction of the mechanics has permitted the joint gradually to improve with time in spite of its initially unpromising appearance.

In Table 8.3 it is seen that 10 hips were treated by means of rotation only at the site of the osteotomy, and 35 by rotation combined with a little varus; while 7, in which there was no evidence of subluxation, were not treated at all. The results in the group where rotation only was carried out are obviously unsatisfactory. If this group is disregarded and the group in which subluxation was corrected by means of rotation combined with varus is compared with the group in which no treatment was carried out because there was no evidence of subluxation, it will be seen that the results are remarkably similar. Although the numbers here are too small to allow any firm

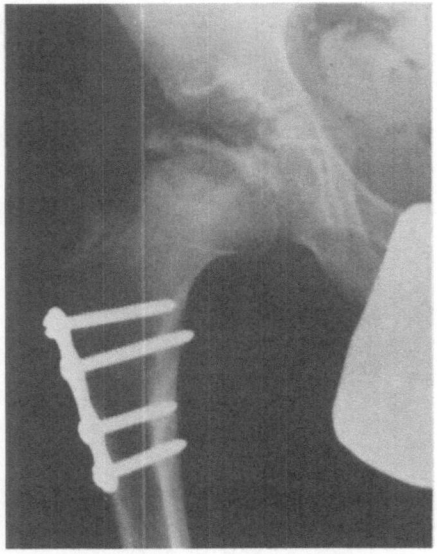

Fig. 8.46. Six months after the radiograph seen in Fig. 8.45 was taken, the appearance suggests that the result will be poor

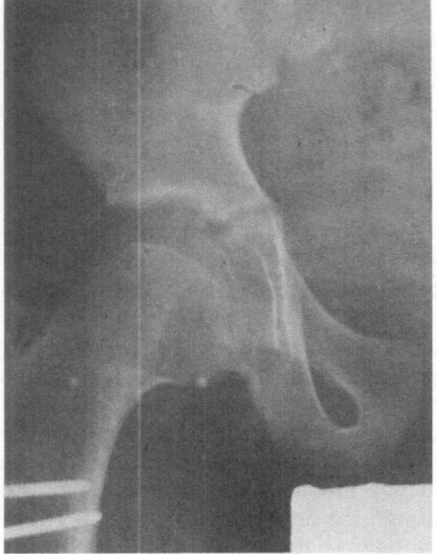

Fig. 8.47. The radiograph 6 years after that seen in Fig. 8.46 shows that the lesion has healed in a much better shape than was anticipated, and further remodelling can be expected to take place for the better

Table 8.3. Results obtained in Perthes' disease

	Results		
	Good	Fair	Poor
Rotation only Total 10	3 (30%)	3 (30%)	4 (40%)
Rotation and varus[a] Total 35	30 (86%)	4 (11.4%)	1 (2.6%)
Untreated (No subluxation) Total 7	6 (85.7%)	0	1 (14%)

[a] In Table 8.3 one hip has been deliberately omitted from those with varus and rotation osteotomies. This is because the hip had developed satisfactorily for more than 5 years when osteochondritis dissecans developed, which was the cause of subsequent deterioration.

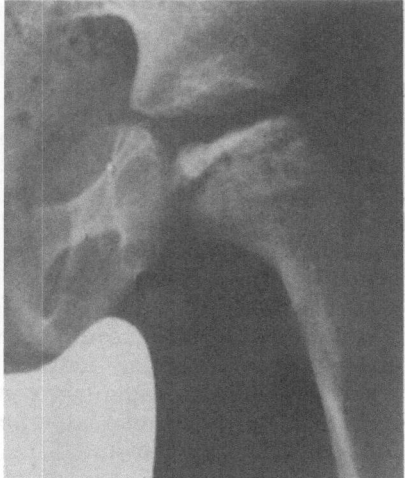

Fig. 8.48. Severe changes in the ossific nucleus in a boy aged 8. Again, the appearance suggests that the metaphysis is involved

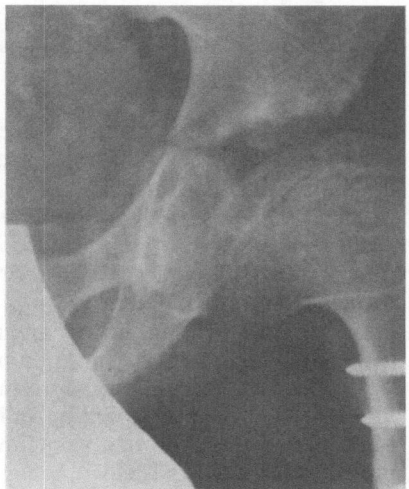

Fig. 8.49. Three years after osteotomy on the hip shown in Fig. 8.48 the result is poor. The head is mushroomed and poorly covered by the acetabulum, although there is no subluxation

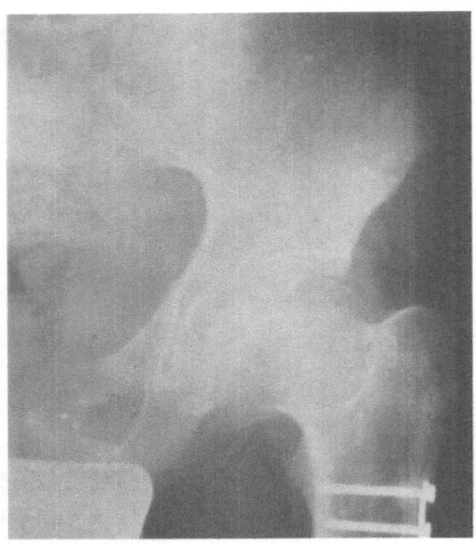

Fig. 8.50. Six years after the radiograph shown in Fig. 8.49 was taken there has been a marked improvement. The femoral head is less flattened and is now adequately covered by the acetabulum. The neck is short because of premature closure of the growth plate

conclusions, the results strongly suggest that in those hips in which there is no subluxation (i.e., either there never was any subluxation or it was adequately corrected at operation) it can be expected that over the years a good result can be obtained in approximately 80% but there will be a further 20% in which the result will be unsatisfactory because of damage done to the growth plate by the initial ischaemia (Glimcher 1977). The degree of failure will depend on the extent to which the growth plate has been affected. Even though the growth plate has been damaged the degree of deformity can be reduced by the elimination of subluxation (Figs. 8.49 and 8.50).

There remains the problem of choosing between bloodless (one can hardly call 3 or 4 years of bed rest or splintage conservative) treatment or surgery. The rationale of treatment can be divided into two groups: (1) relief from weight-bearing; and (2) femoral head containment.

1) *Relief from weight-bearing* can be obtained in a number of different ways—by prolonged recumbency, sitting in a wheelchair, or by calipers, slings or other appliances. Evans and Lloyd-Roberts (1958), comparing the different methods, were of the opinion that there was little to choose between them and the results of treatment were very little better than the results of doing nothing. They summed up by saying "... we may say that we were comparing one useless method with another". The present author agrees with this whole-heartedly.

2) *Femoral head containment* can be obtained by external splintage as first practised by A. O. Parker (McKibbin 1975) in Cardiff and Oswestry in the 1920s (see p. 155). This was then modified by Petrie and Bitenc (1971). This method allowed a certain amount of ambulation. Both these techniques produced good results because they removed the deforming factor, i.e., the subluxation. Unfortunately both involve the child being partially or completely immobolised for several years of his childhood, and it is still unknown how much damage is done to other joints, particularly the knees, during this prolonged period of enforced splintage.

Surgical treatment aims to do just the same and if it produced results which were no better than containment by splintage it would still have the enormous advantage of involving the child in a very limited period of immobility which rarely exceeds 3 months and is often less.

COMMENT

A critical review of the development of the hips in these two series, of congenital dislocation of the hip and Perthes' disease, emphasises how the development of the hip joint and the shape of its component parts is influenced by the mechanics of the joint. Eccentric movement, however slight, leads to progressive deterioration, but restoration of concentric movement restores normal development. But the two conditions behave quite differently. In congenital dislocation it is more difficult to establish concentric movement and once established, eccentric movement may well redevelop. This can happen at any age, even in hips which were previously normal. Many hips which develop arthritis in middle life have an appearance suggesting that the cause was dysplasia. Careful examination of the radiograph shows that the dew-drop on the medial wall of the acetabulum is thin, as in a normal hip. If there had been dysplasia during the growth period the dew-drop would have been much thickened; this shows that the displacement must have taken place after the cessation of growth.

While in the congenitally displaced hip there is a very strong tendency for the treated hip to deteriorate (Muller and Seddon 1953), a fact which would be supported by most orthopaedic surgeons who treat the condition in any numbers, in Perthes' disease just the reverse seems to be the case. Once concentric movement has been established (or in those cases where it was never lost) improvement in the shape of the joint will continue for a great many years, well beyond the cessation of growth; and there is very little if any tendency to relapse unless some condition such as osteochondritis dissecans should develop (Ratcliff 1967b). Even when severe deformity has developed deterioration is slow and symptoms may not develop before late middle life, as was shown by Ratcliff (1956, 1967a). The author has seen a patient who had gross Perthes' disease who served for 20 years in the British Army and ran the 4000 metres for the Army. He was seen at the age of 43 because of the development of a loose body in the joint. Apart from this he had no symptoms and never knew there was anything wrong with the joint.

Why should there be this difference between Perthes' disease, in which despite severe deformity there is little disability and symptoms are long delayed, and congenital dislocation, where the deformity may be much less marked, the deterioration is rapid, and severe symptoms develop early? Perhaps it is because in Perthes' disease as the hip develops the acetabulum adapts to the deformity of the femoral head, producing a horizontal joint which is stable and in which some sort of concentric movement develops in spite of the deformity, whereas in the congenitally displaced hip instability with an eccentric type of movement readily develops. Again, why should a stable hip, even though severely deformed, last a long time without giving trouble while an unstable hip rapidly deteriorates?

Perhaps articular cartilage will only stand up to the one type of movement for which it is designed. In the hip this is a rotational movement whichever way the hip is moved but if a sliding, i.e. eccentric, type of movement develops it rapidly degenerates. While this is pure conjecture it seems to fit many of the facts. If this mechanism applies to the hip it must surely apply to every joint in the body.

REFERENCES

Axer A (1965) Subtrochanteric osteotomy in the treatment of Perthes' disease. J Bone Joint Surg [Br] 47:489

Axer, A, Sculler MG, Segal D, Rzetelny V, Gershuni-Gordon DH (1973) Subtrochanteric osteotomy in the treatment of Legg-Calvé-Perthes' syndrome. Acta Orthop Scand 44:31

Boldero J, Kemp HBS (1966) Radiological changes in Perthes' disease. Br J Radiol 39:744

Catterall A (1971) The natural history of Perthes' disesase. J Bone Joint Surg [Br] 53:37

Evans DL, Lloyd-Roberts GC (1958) Treatment of Legg-Calvé-Perthes' disease: A comparison of in-patient and out-patient treatment. J Bone Joint Surg [Br] 40:182

Glimcher MJ (1977) Biological, geometrical and anatomical considerations of the pathophysiology and treatment of Legg-Calvé-Perthes' disease. Proceedings of the First International Symposium on Legg-Calvé-Perthes' Syndrome, Nov 17–18, p 8

Kemp HBS (1973) Perthes' disease. An experimental and clinical study. Ann R Coll Surg Engl 52:18

Lauritzen J (1975) Legg-Calvé-Perthes' disease. Acta Orthop Scand [Suppl] 159

Legg AT (1910) An obscure affection of the hip joint. Boston Medical and Surgical Journal 162:202

McKibbin B (1975) Recent developments in Perthes' disease. Churchill Livingstone, London (Recent advances in orthopaedics, p 173)

McKibbin B, Rallis Z (1974) Pathological changes in a case of Perthes' disease. J Bone Joint Surg [Br] 56:438

Muller GM, Seddon HJ (1953) Late results of treatment of congenital dislocation of the hip. J Bone Joint Surg [Br] 35:342

Petrie JG, Bitenc I (1971) The abduction weight-bearing treatment in Legg-Calvé-Perthes' disease. J Bone Joint Surg [Br] 53:54

Ratliff AHC (1956) Pseudocoxalgia. J Bone Joint Surg [Br] 38:498

Ratliff AHC (1967a) Perthes' disease. A study of 34 hips observed for 30 years. J Bone Joint Surg [Br] 49:102

Ratliff AHC (1967b) Osteochondritis dissecans following Legg-Calvé-Perthes' disease. J Bone Joint Surg [Br] 49:108

Salter RB (1966a) Experimental and clinical aspects of Perthes' disease. J Bone Joint Surg [Br] 48:393

Salter RB (1966b) Legg-Perthes' disease. J Bone Joint Surg [Br] 48:854

Sanchis M, Zahir A, Freeman MAR (1973) The experimental simulation of Perthes' disease by consecutive interruptions of the blood supply to the capital femoral epiphysis in the puppy. J Bone Joint Surg [Am] 55:335

Somerville EW (1971) Perthes' disease of the hip. J Bone Joint Surg [Br] 53:639

Somerville EW (1980) Perthes' disease Acta Orthop Belg 46:399

Trueta J (1957) The normal vascular anatomy of the human femoral head during growth. J Bone Joint Surg [Br] 39:358

Trueta J, Harrison MHM (1953) Normal vascular anatomy of the femoral head in adult man. J Bone Joint Surg [Br] 35:442

9 Persistent Foetal Alignment

Typical congenital dislocation of the hip may be a disease entity in itself, but it is closely allied to variants in the shape of the upper end of the femur. The importance of anteversion has already been emphasised. Since it plays such a large part in the development of displacement, in its persistence, and in its recurrence, it seems pertinent to include a chapter on the problem.

DEFORMITY

Primary

Anteversion is the angle at which the neck of the femur projects forwards in relation to the rest of the femur. This does not suggest that it is projecting forwards from an otherwise normal upper end of the femur. The upper end of a femur with 45° of anteversion seen in isolation from the rest of the femur looks like the upper end of a femur in which the angle is normal. It is likely that the angle is produced by a torsion in the inter- or subtrochanteric regions.

At the time of birth the angle of anteversion may vary widely. In the majority it will be about 25°–30° but it may be as little as nil or as much as 45°, and occasionally a little more. In most cases it will have moulded to 5°–10°, which is normal, by the completion of growth. In some the moulding will have been less than this and in some no remodelling will have taken place at all. The relationship between this condition and congenital dislocation of the hip is shown diagrammatically in Fig. 1.6. It has been found that in 20% of patients with unilateral displacement of the hip an excessive degree of anteversion has persisted in the other hip. Since anteversion is moulded away in the majority of cases, for it to persist in 20% in any one group suggests that the initial incidence must have been very high. While anteversion is not the cause of displacement it is an important factor. A child with an excessive degree of anteversion is more likely to develop displacement than one where the angle is less.

It is difficult to measure the angle of anteversion in a very young child radiologically, but it can be measured clinically once full extension has been achieved. In the normal hip the arc of rotation with the hip fully extended is 45° medial and 45° lateral; with 45° of anteversion the arc is 90° medial and 0° lateral, because as far as the hip is concerned anteversion and lateral rotation are the same thing; with the leg in neutral rotation clinically, the upper end of the femur will be in full lateral rotation so that further lateral rotation will not be possible unless the anterior part of the capsule is stretched. With the hip in flexion anteversion has no effect on the arc of rotation (Figs. 9.1–9.3).

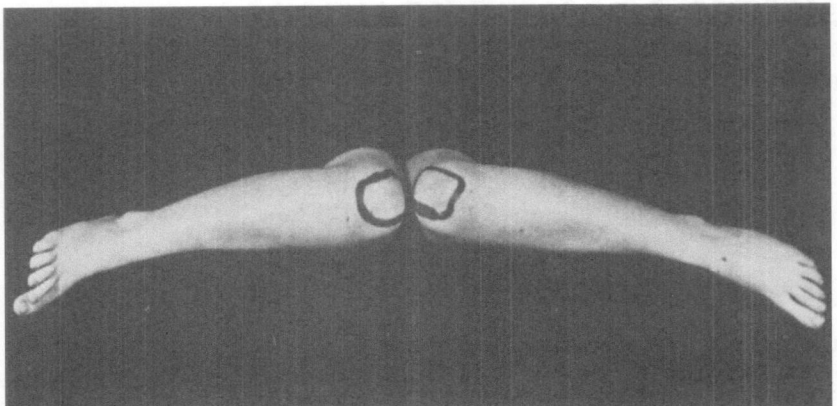

Fig. 9.1. These hips are in full extension with 90° of medial rotation

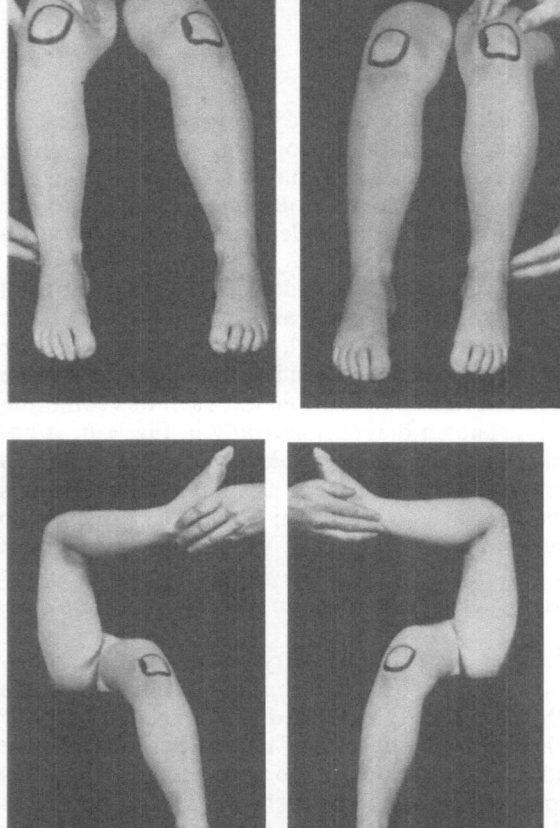

Fig. 9.2. With the hips in extension no lateral rotation is possible

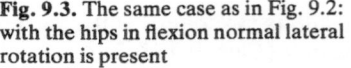

Fig. 9.3. The same case as in Fig. 9.2: with the hips in flexion normal lateral rotation is present

Secondary

When starting to walk, a high proportion of children turn their feet medially. This is physiological and usually of no significance; in a short while most children will walk normally, but there is a proportion in whom the intoeing is due to structural changes. In some it will be due to medial torsion of the tibia, which is often a legacy from a previous bowing which has spontaneously corrected, and in others it will be due to persistence of an excessive degree of anteversion of the neck of the femur, or as it may be called persistent foetal alignment of the hip. It is in this group that further trouble may arise.

In some of these the angle of anteversion may be gradually moulded away as shown by the progressive development of lateral rotation, and if this is sufficient the legs will develop normally, but if this moulding has not started by the age of 5 years it is unlikely to do so (Harris 1972) and in this case one of several things may happen.

1) The child will walk normally and there will never be any disability or secondary deformity;

2) The child will continue to walk with an intoeing gait but no secondary deformity will develop because there will be no deforming force;

3) The child will cease to intoe and will put the foot down squarely on the ground with the toes to the front, but when weight is borne the knee will turn medially with every stride. This places a lateral torsional strain on the leg below the knee and a pronating force on the foot, flattening it onto the ground. With time this will cause the development of a twist of the tibia or flattening of the foot, and sometimes both. If the foot is strong most of the strain will fall on the tibia, and while it is growing and malleable it will develop a lateral twist. The degree of torsion which develops is usually 15°–20° and only exceptionally will it be more. In many cases this will be associated with medial bowing of the upper end of the tibia. This is clinically very similar to tibia vara, but no epiphyseal changes have been seen (Figs. 9.4 and 9.5).

If the foot is hypermobile the strain falling on it will cause it to become increasingly flat and valgus. In doing so it will to some extent cushion the strain on the tibia, so that at times all the secondary deformity will be in the foot. The commonest deformity is a well-marked lateral torsion of the tibia with a minor degree of valgus of the foot.

There is no doubt at all that this condition is a true entity, but there is still some disagreement as to whether it should be treated or not, and if it should be treated— how?

TREATMENT

Rationale

It is often said that this condition will resolve if left alone. This is certainly so in many very young children, and it is likely that it passes unnoticed in many more. A follow-up of many children has shown that if no lateral rotation has developed by the age of 5 or 6 years it is very unlikely to. If, however, some degree of lateral rotation is developing by this age it is quite possible that there will be further improvement, and the child should be watched without treatment unless or until secondary deformities are appearing, when surgery should be undertaken without undue delay. In some cases the decision presents no problem but there are many which are borderline. There are three factors to be taken into consideration: (1) function; (2) cosmesis; and (3) arthritis.

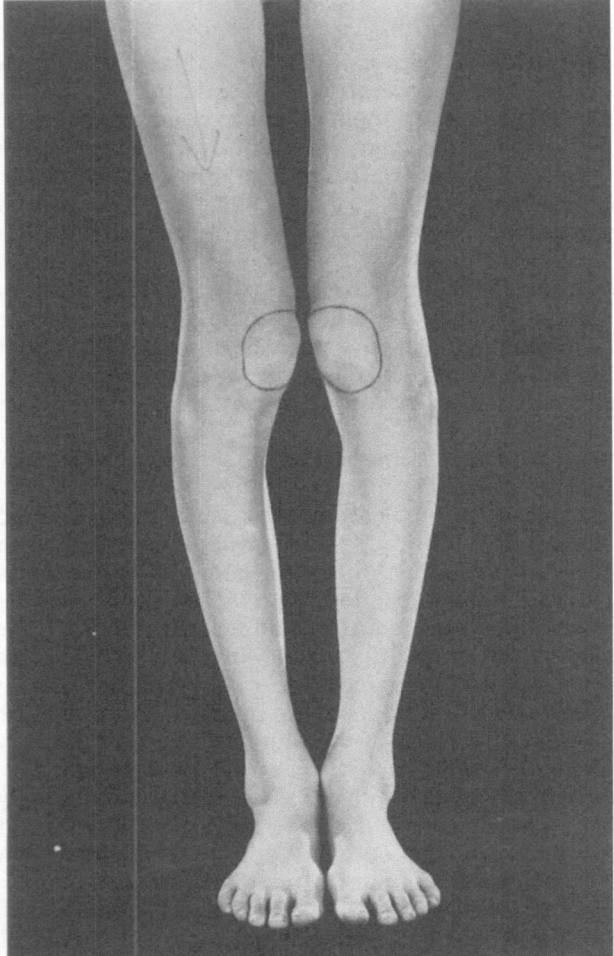

Fig. 9.4. Typical deformity of persistent foetal alignment, seen when the child stands with the feet together

FUNCTION

An intoeing gait is in no way inconsistent with normal activity. In fact, it is well recognised that many athletes have this form of gait. But in the athlete the intoeing is either postural or due to medial torsion of the tibia, in both of which conditions the axis of the knee is normal. In persistent foetal alignment the knees are turned in towards each other when the feet are together, so that the axis of the knee is at an angle to that of the ankle joint causing the feet to be thrown out to the sides during running; this is not generally consistent with athletic ability. Persistent foetal alignment does not always cause clumsiness but a frequent comment from relatives and the patient is that agility has greatly improved since correction.

COSMESIS

This condition is more important in girls than in boys. The deformity is ugly, and

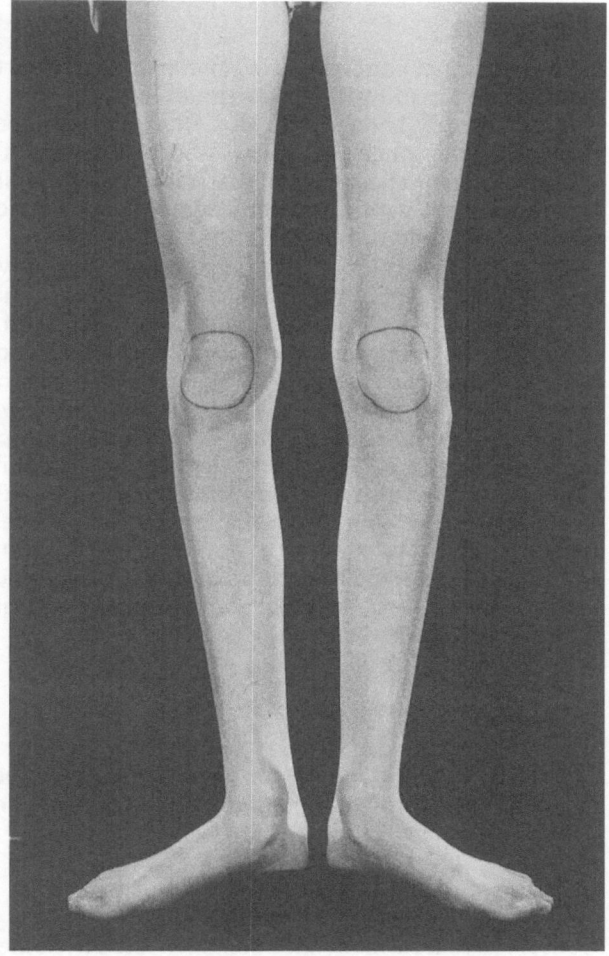

Fig. 9.5. The deformity in persistent foetal alignment looks slightly better when the child stands with the legs fully laterally rotated and the feet at 90° to each other

sometimes very ugly (Figs. 9.4 and 9.5), and some children have been mistakenly diagnosed as being spastic. Children rarely complain when young; it is the relatives who ask advice. In explaining the condition it must not be forgotten that the ugliness will increase as secondary changes develop, and when boy friends become an important factor in their lives this may present a big problem. By this time, instead of only a femoral osteotomy being required, the torsional changes in the tibia will need correction as well; an added complication which could have been avoided.

In many cases the decision is difficult and after explaining the problem it is usually wise to send the parents and child away to think it over and then discuss the whole thing again 3 or 4 months later.

While treatment of this condition may be approached with some scepticism by some orthopaedic surgeons, there is no doubt about its popularity with patients and parents. This is one of the operations for which the orthopaedic surgeon constantly receives thanks.

ARTHRITIS

Is this rotational abnormality a precursor of osteoarthritis, and if so of which joint? The question is still without a definite answer.

It has already been shown that there is a connection between persistent foetal alignment and congenital dislocation of the hip. Although anteversion is not the cause of congenital displacement it has a bearing on the mechanism of dislocation, so that those born with a greater degree of anteversion than 25° are more liable to displacement than those born with less.

The excessive angle of anteversion may persist without displacement occurring, but the mechanism of displacement will still be present. Just because displacement has not occurred early does not mean that it will not develop later, causing an eccentric type of movement which will inevitably lead to arthritis. Many arthritic hips show evidence of subluxation but there is no evidence of previous dysplasia, and the dew-drop will be thin, clear evidence that there was no displacement during the period of growth. It seems that while there is no certain evidence that persistent foetal alignment of the hip predisposes to osteoarthritis of the hip this must be suspected. It may also be a factor in osteoarthritis of the knee because of the torsional strain and the bowing of the upper end of the tibia, both of which could cause an eccentric type of movement to develop. The foot must also be at risk. The torsional strain imposed on the foot in the presence of persistent foetal alignment is sufficient to cause flattening of the arch, and it would be surprising if it did not in the long term do some lasting damage to the joints.

Techniques

The initial object of any form of treatment must be the correction of the primary rotational deformity of the femur before the secondary changes have become established.

CONSERVATIVE

Conservative treatment has been advocated by some surgeons. This involves the use of external rotational night splints and/or twister braces worn during the day. Such forcible rotation has nothing to commend it; all it will do is ensure the development of the secondary deformities without correcting the primary. If treatment is to be undertaken it must be surgical.

SURGICAL

The most important correction which must always be done is that of the primary deformity in the femur. All that is required is to produce a good range of lateral rotation at the hip when the hip is in full extension—ideally 45°. This is done by a simple rotation osteotomy, the technique for which has already been described on p. 52. Both femurs are operated on at the same operation, and if the correction has been carried out before the secondary deformities have developed they will not develop. If they have already developed to a minor degree they can often be ignored and may well correct spontaneously once the deforming force has been removed, particularly in the young child. If the secondary deformities have become established they will not correct spontaneously and will need to be corrected surgically. This will involve an osteotomy of the tibia to produce medial rotation. The amount of lateral torsion of the tibia is usually quite small, and it is rarely necessary to rotate the tibia medially at the osteotomy by more than 15°–20°. If varus is present this will need to be corrected at the same time.

The technique of tibial osteotomy is quite different from osteotomy of the femur, because while the femur is round the tibia is triangular with flat surfaces.

The subcutaneous surface of the tibia is exposed in its upper third through a straight incision about 10 cm in length. The bone is exposed subperiosteally all round. The muscles on the lateral side should never be retracted with a bone lever because of the risk of producing an anterior compartment syndrome, small though it may be. The bone is divided exactly transversely; first a small drill is used and the division is then completed with a thin osteotome. If it is necessary to correct a varus deformity at the same time as rotation it will be necessary to divide the fibula also, but rotation up to 25° alone can be performed without this.

The osteotomy is fixed with a four-screw plate which has previously been twisted to the required angle and angled as necessary to correct the varus. The periosteum is closed over the plate with a continuous suture and the wound is closed. Figure 9.6 shows the correction of one leg before the second came to operation. Before operation the two legs were identical.

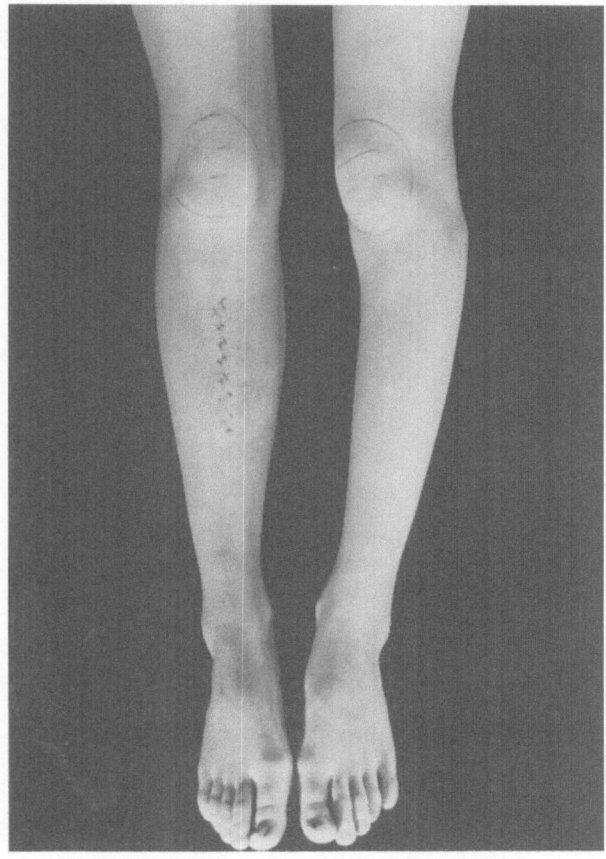

Fig. 9.6. The right leg after correction of persistent foetal alignment. The left leg has not yet been corrected. The improvement is striking

The operation is very often carried out bilaterally in two stages, the femur and tibia in one leg being operated on the same day and the other leg being operated on 1 or 2 weeks later. The most difficult part of the operation is ensuring that the two legs will look identical afterwards.

Postoperatively the osteotomies are protected in a hip spica. The operation can incorporate the use of heavy-duty plate with six or eight screws, with the object of being able to dispense with plaster altogether. Whatever is used for internal fixation will not permit weight-bearing in safety, so the only gain is in mobilisation. In this age group mobilisation has presented no problem after plaster, and it is only in cases where plaster has not been used that any complications have been encountered.

Occasionally the foot deformity will be sufficiently severe—in that it will be flat and in valgus—to be a liability. In such cases it should be stabilised with the heel in the mid-position (never varus) by means of the Grice–Green operation on the subtalar joint. In all the cases where this has been done the results have been most satisfactory.

Following removal of the plaster mobilisation will take place reasonably quickly, but the child will always walk badly at first and the parents must be warned of this in advance. The length of time for which the child will walk badly will depend very much on the age at the time of operation. At the age of 5, normal walking should have been achieved within 2–3 months, but if the child is over the age of 14 years it may take as long as a year, which is obviously another good reason for early operation.

REFERENCES

Harris NH (1972) Rotational deformities and their secondary effects in the lower extremities in children. J Bone Joint Surg [Br] 54:172
Somerville EW (1957) Persistent foetal alignment of the hip. J Bone Joint Surg [Br] 39:106

10 Development of the Upper End of the Femur

From what has already been said it should be clear that the development of the upper end of the femur must play an important part in the way in which the hip joint develops both in health and in disease. There is a further condition, congenital coxa vara, which throws light on the way in which this development takes place and warrants consideration.

AETIOLOGY

The blood supply to the original cartilaginous anlage of the femur in utero is via the nutrient artery which enters about the middle of the shaft. Here it forms an ossific nucleus and divides into ascending and descending branches, which progress towards the ends of the bone, carrying the ossification with them. By the time of birth the ossification will have reached about to the base of the neck of the femur (Trueta 1957). It continues to extend until an epiphyseal line is formed between it and the epiphyses, forming a metaphysis which extends from the medial side of the head to the lateral side of the greater trochanter. It is from this rather complicated growth plate that growth takes place at the proximal end of the femur. Orderly growth must depend very much on the local blood supply and should this be damaged abnormalities of growth will necessarily result.

The normal pattern of development is shown diagrammatically in Fig. 10.1. It can be seen that orderly ossification has taken place, accompanied by the ascending blood vessel up to the epiphysis which extends from the medial side of the head to the lateral side of the great trochanter. If there had been an interruption to the ascending vessel before it reached the epiphysis ossification would be halted at the same level and there would be no possibility of orderly growth from below (Fig. 10.2). This is a severe type of congenital coxa vara, and in a radiograph taken at birth it could be mistaken for a congenital absence of the upper end of the femur (Fig. 10.3). But if the hip is watched over a number of years it will be seen that an ossific nucleus develops in the femoral head, which is in the acetabulum (Fig. 10.4). An arthrogram of the hip seen in Fig. 10.4 shows that the acetabulum was within normal limits and there was an apparently normal head in it. It also suggested that there was a neck (Fig. 10.5). Five years later (Fig. 10.6) it can be seen that the head of the femur had undergone complete ossification, the gap between the head and the shaft was becoming filled with irregular bone, and the great tronchanter was beginning to appear. This is because the head and the great trochanter have a blood supply of their own and are not dependent on the nutrient artery. The intervening gap is filled with irregular bone which has developed from perichondral vessels. Clearly there is no way in which a metaphysis could form and therefore there can be no growth. A similar case picked up at this stage (Fig. 10.7) was operated on by my colleague Mr. R. G. Taylor, who

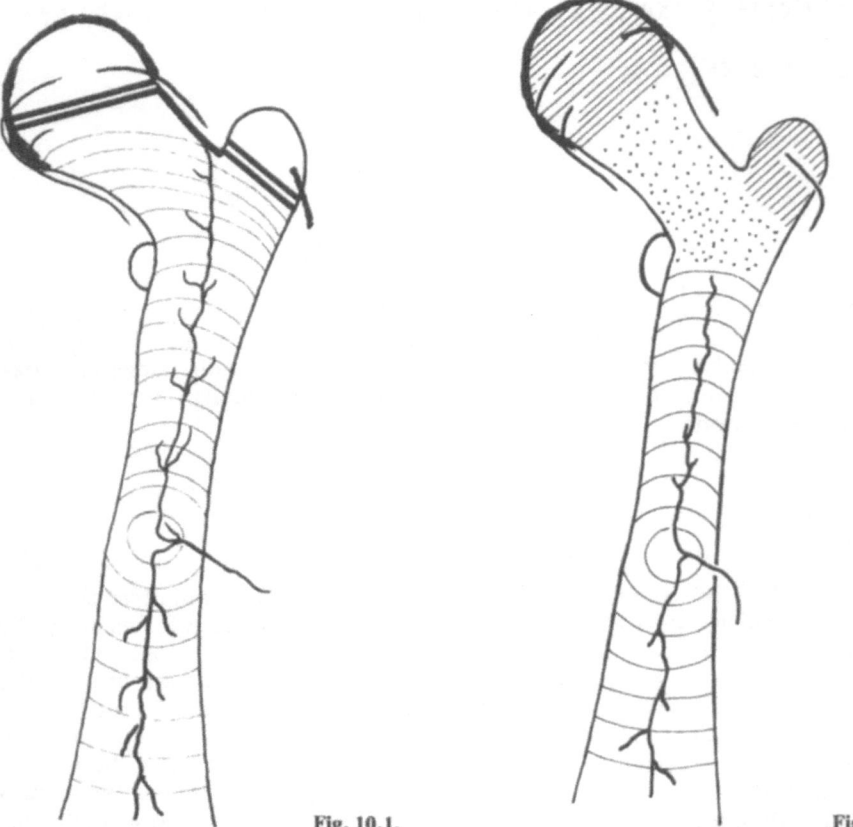

Fig. 10.1.   Fig. 10.2.

Fig. 10.1. Normal pattern of blood supply in relation to the ossification of the upper end of the femur. It also shows the relation between the articular surface of the head of the femur and the epiphysis. On the medial side a small portion of the head lies distal to the epiphyseal line and has the same blood supply as the head (Trueta 1957)

Fig. 10.2. Situation when the blood supply to the metaphysis via the nutrient artery is interrupted at a low level. There is still a normal blood supply to the head and great trochanter

performed a high femoral valgus osteotomy. The whole of the upper end of the femur fused into one piece of bone with no evidence of epiphysis or metaphysis, so that no growth was possible at this end of the femur (Fig. 10.8).

The first case mentioned above (Fig. 10.3) was operated on at the age of 8 months, when the nucleus of the head was first seen. At operation a cartilaginous upper end of the femur was clearly seen, which was joined to the bony shaft by fibrous union only. A bone graft taken from lower down the shaft was placed across the pseudarthrosis in the vain hope that orderly ossification might be restored. The operation was a failure, as it was in two other patients with similar conditions. But the operative findings support the views already expressed regarding the nature of this condition (Lloyd-Roberts and Stone 1963). In this particular case there was a history of trauma. The mother had fallen down stairs in the seventh month of pregnancy and injured her abdomen. The injury was such that she was taken to hospital at once because it was feared she might lose the baby. But there is no proof that trauma was the cause of the damage, and it is unusual to obtain a history of trauma in such cases. All that can be said is that anything which causes an interruption of the ascending blood supply could produce this type of lesion.

If the defect occurred at a slightly higher level at the base of the neck (Fig. 10.9) a normal epiphysis would develop in the trochanter with a normal epiphyseal line where growth can take place. But the head and neck can never have a metaphysis and so these parts could not grow. This must inevitably result in the development of a gross coxa vara, which is more typical of congenital coxa vara. The trochanter continues to grow but the head and neck are left behind (Fig. 10.10). At first an apparent gap is seen in the neck but it is cartilage; even without treatment ossification takes place from the perichondral vessels but with severe deformity (Fig. 10.11).

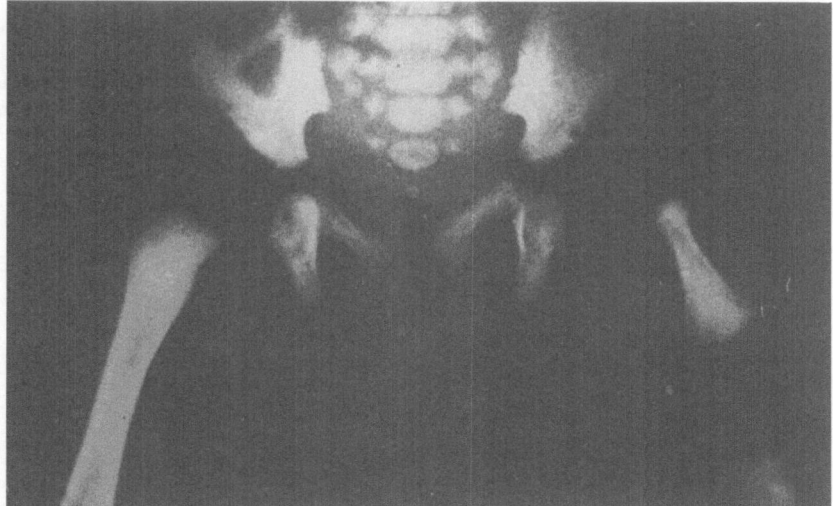

Fig. 10.3. Severe coxa vara on the left compared with a normal hip on the right

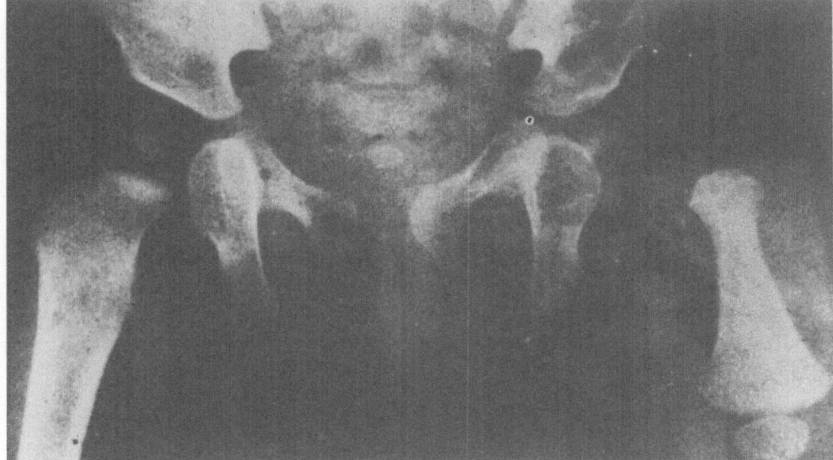

Fig. 10.4. Nine months after the radiograph shown in Fig. 10.3 was taken an ossific nucleus is visible in the femoral head, which is well placed in the acetabulum

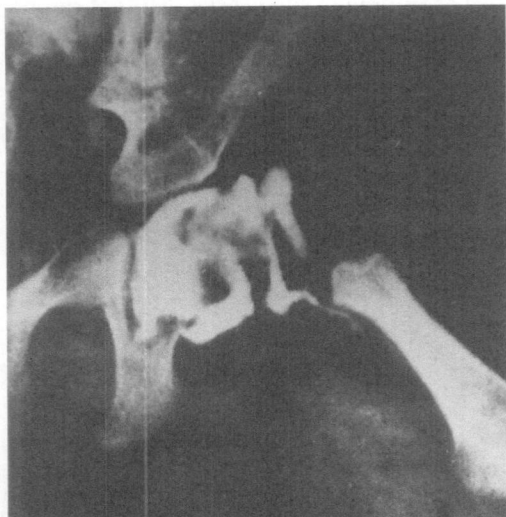

Fig. 10.5. An arthrogram shows a
surprisingly normal-looking femoral
head. It also suggests that the upper end
of the femur is present

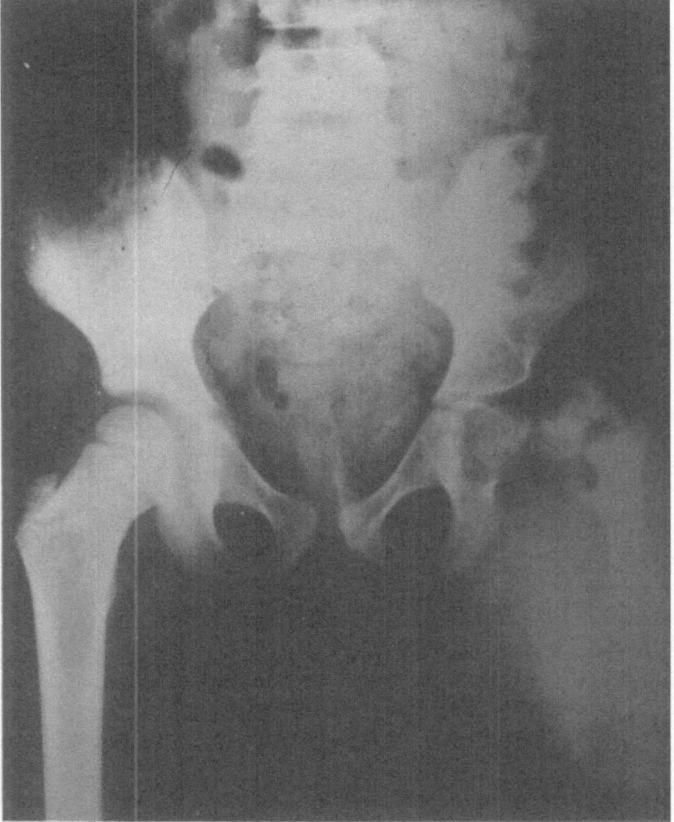

Fig. 10.6. Five years after the arthrogram shown in Fig. 10.5 was taken, the femoral head is fully ossified,
the greater trochanter is partially ossified, and there is patchy ossification in the rest of the upper end,
which never had a proper blood supply

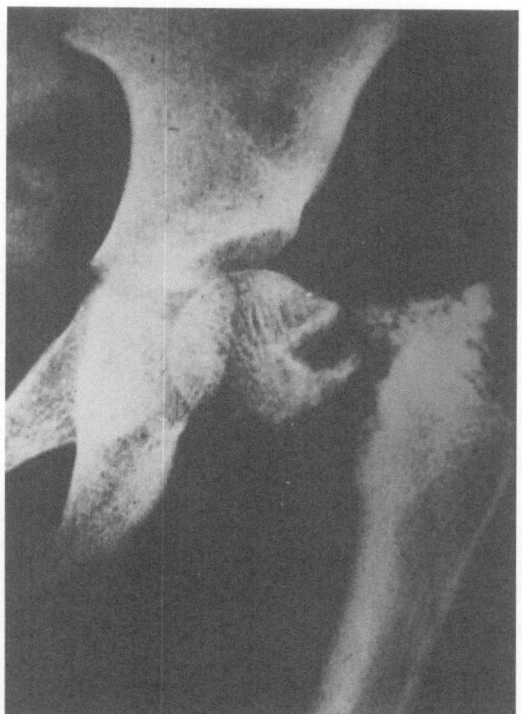

Fig. 10.7. Radiograph showing an identical case to that of Figs. 10.4–10.6 at a later stage

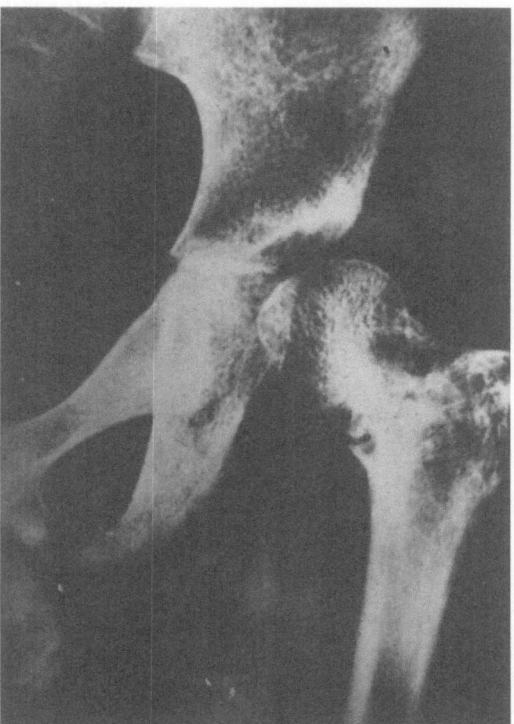

Fig. 10.8. After correction of the deformity shown in Fig. 10.7 the whole of the upper end is now bone, with no sign of a metaphysis

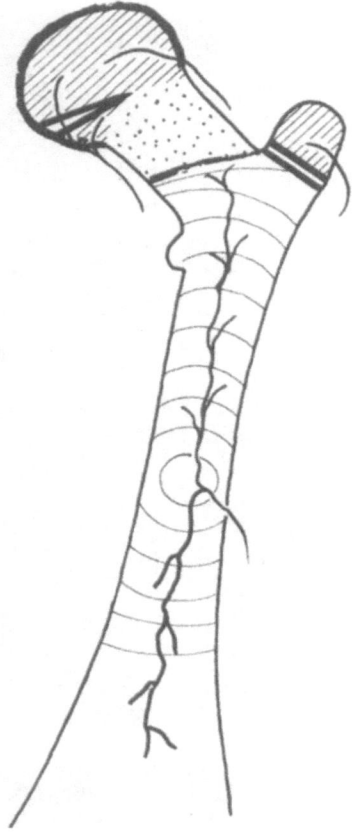

Fig. 10.9. When the interruption to the nutrient artery is higher than in the cases shown in Figs. 10.4–10.6 and Figs. 10.7 and 10.8, as is seen in this drawing an epiphyseal line and metaphysis can develop in relation to the great trochanter

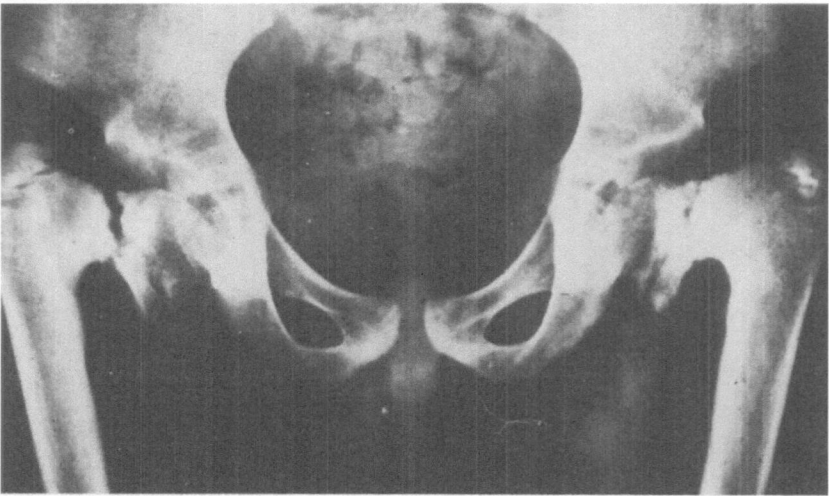

Fig. 10.10. A radiograph showing the condition illustrated in the previous drawing. The great trochanters have grown normally, leaving the head behind. There is a small gap still ununited. The separate triangular piece of bone is clearly seen below the head

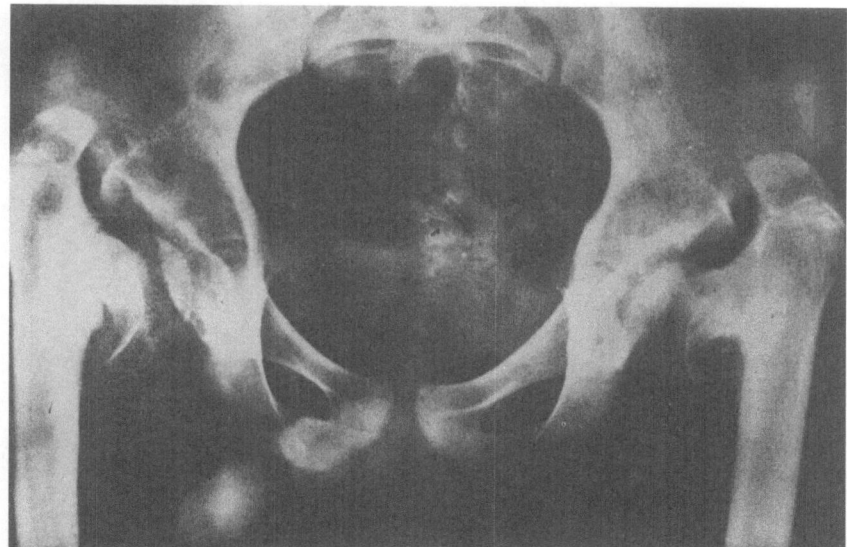

Fig. 10.11. Ossification is complete without treatment

In the radiographs shown in Figs. 10.10 and 10.12 a fragment of bone can be seen which is separated from the capital epiphysis and from the neck. In the literature this has often been referred to as the 'triangular fragment', which is a constant feature of this condition (Blockey 1969; Elmslie 1913; Fairbanks 1928).

This fragment can be explained following study of the vascular pattern (Trueta 1957). The head of the femur is that part of the upper end of the femur which is covered with articular cartilage. This is not the same as the epiphysis, because on the medial side the articular cartilage extends distal to the epiphyseal line. The vascular supply is to the head of the femur and not just to the epiphysis (Fig. 10.9), so that there is a small area of bone distal to the epiphyseal line on the medial side which derives its blood supply from the circumflex artery and not from the nutrient artery. Between this piece of bone and the epiphysis there is a small gap, which is all that is left of the epiphyseal line. It is of no practical significance and disappears when growth ceases.

TREATMENT

There is no useful surgical treatment for the correction of the most severe degree of this condition, as described at the beginning of this chapter, and it is necessary to have recourse to some prosthesis, poor though these may be. But those in which the deformity is less severe can be helped considerably by means of a suitable osteotomy (Fig. 10.12). Whatever type of osteotomy is used the deformity must be over-corrected (Fig. 10.13). This is a growth deformity and will continue to recur until growth ceases. For this reason, where the deformity is severe it may be necessary to repeat the procedure more than once.

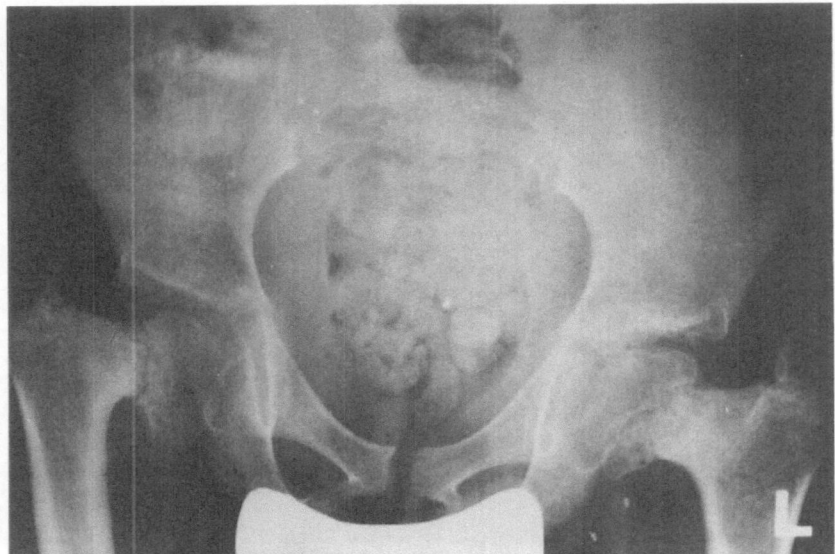

Fig. 10.12. A similar lesion to that seen in Fig. 10.10, but less severe

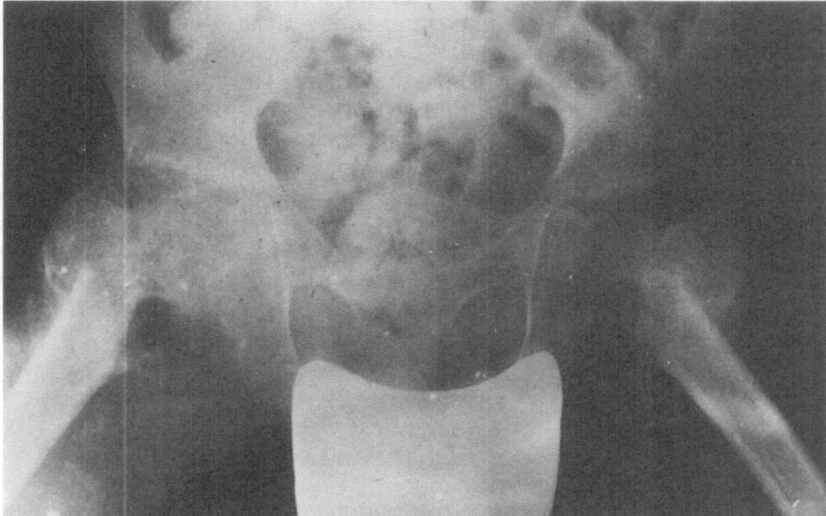

Fig. 10.13. Same patient as in Fig. 10.11. Corrective osteotomies with wide abduction

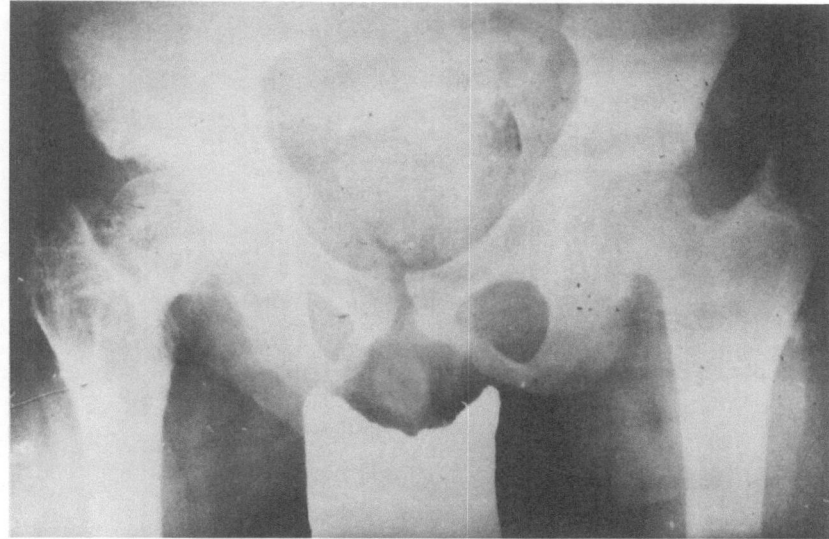

Fig. 10.14. Same patient as in Figs. 10.12 and 10.13. The final position at the age of 17. No further deformity will occur because growth has ceased

REFERENCES

Blockey NJ (1969) Observations on congenital coxa vara. J Bone Joint Surg [Br] 51:106

Elmslie RC (1913) Congenital coxa vara: Its pathology and treatment. Hodder & Stoughton, London

Fairbank HAT (1928) Infantile coxa vara. In: Robert Jones birthday volume. University Press, Oxford, p 225

Lloyd-Roberts GC, Stone KH (1963) Congenital hypoplasia of the upper femur. J Bone Joint Surg [Br] 45:557

Morgan JD, Somerville EW (1960) Normal and abnormal development of the upper end of the femur. J Bone Joint Surg [Br] 42:264

Trueta J (1957) The normal vascular anatomy of the human femoral head during growth. J Bone Joint Surg [Br] 39:611

Subject Index

M. K. Dalinka

Arthrography

1980. 324 figures, 4 tables. XIV, 209 pages
(Comprehensive Manuals in Radiology)
ISBN 3-540-90466-2

Arthrography – the radiological examination of joints after the injection of a contrast material – is one of the most active areas in the new subspecialty of interventional diagnostics. This book is a complete evaluation of the use of arthrography in all applicable joints of the human body. Outstandingly illustrated, it covers the knee, ankle, hip, wrist, elbow, and temporomandibular articulation, as well as other joints and bursae. Each chapter includes normal anatomy and variations, description of technique, normal and pathological arthrography findings, and the clinical significance of arthrography in each joint. Special consideration is given to the use of arthrography in children.
The extensive and up-to-date literature included in this beautifully written work will make it both a valuable reference for practicing radiologists, as well as a comprehensive introduction to the discipline for residents.

J. L. Gwinn, P. Stanley

Diagnostic Imaging in Pediatric Trauma

With contribution by numerous experts

1980. 275 figures in 468 separate illustrations,
7 tables. XIII, 199 pages
(Current Diagnostic Pediatrics)
ISBN 3-540-09473-3

Trauma to various organ systems is a common medical problem in the pediatric age group. The increase in vehicular traffic, active participation in contact sports, and a changing social atmosphere have brought with them a sharp rise in the incidence of injury to children. This book concentrates on radiologic methods for the diagnosis of childhood injuries. Special attention is paid to how pediatric trauma differs from that in the adult. The material is for the most part, based on case histories from Children's Hospital Los Angeles, to which the authors add their own considerable experience in the area. The book is divided into the various organ systems for easy reference, with pertinent literature included in the bibliography at the end of each chapter. A section on ultrasound and nuclear medicine is included, covering the use of these modalities, where indicated, in all types of trauma.

G. M. Bedbrook

The Care and Management of Spinal Cord Injuries

Foreword by R. W. Jackson

1981. 147 figures. XVI, 351 pages
ISBN 3-540-90494-8

The care and management of patients with spinal cord injuries is a difficult task requiring the team effort of medical and allied health professionals. In this book, G. M. Bedbrook, a noted specialist with many years' experience in the area, provides the practical information a team effort needs for the successful day-to-day handling of such injuries. Carefully organized in an easily accessible format, *The Care and Management of Spinal Cord Injuries* covers all aspects of the diagnosis, treatment and rehabilitation of these patients. A chapter on the paraplegic in developng countries is included, showing that improvement in care can be achieved even with limited resources. An appendix lists suppliers of equipment covered in the book, and important references to the literature are provided at the end of each chapter. Chapters on anatomy, physiology and pathology enable readers to solve practical problems that may arise and can be used as a basic for further reading. All members of the medical team – physicians, surgeons, nurses, and physicians and occupational therapists – will find this book an invaluable reference for optimal care of paraplegics and tetraplegics.

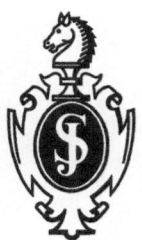

Springer-Verlag
Berlin
Heidelberg
New York

F. Pauwels

Biomechanics of the Locomotor Apparatus

Contributions on the Functional Anatomy of the Locomotor Apparatus

Translated from the German, Completely Revised and Enlarged, Including Seven New Chapters
Translated by P. Maquet, R. Furlong
1980. 733 figures, 22 tables. VIII, 518 pages
ISBN 3-540-09131-9

This classical work of functional anatomy results from more than forty years of study on the adaptation of the human locomotor apparatus to its specific funtion. It was first published in German in 1965. The present edition includes seven additional chapters.
The author analyses the static and dynamic forces acting on the locomotor apparatus and the stresses which they evoke in the tissues. He observes and explains how living tissues react to these stresses. He demonstrates that stretching leads to the formation of connective tissue. Formation of cartilage requires hydrostatic pressure and formation of bone requires immobility of osteogenic tissue. Remodelling of bone depends on the magnitude of the stresses and leads to a trajectorial structure of cancellous bony tissue. These concepts revolutionize the theories previously accepted. Moreover, the author describes how to modify the stresses arising in the tissues in order to achieve therapeutic effects. In this way, he was the first to give a logical solution to the problem of the fractured neck of femur. The concepts of Pauwels are clear. They are confirmed by clinical examples and by histological, anatomical and pathological preparations. They provide the basis for a logical and scientific approach to orthopaedic surgery.

D. I. Abramson, D. S. Miller

Vascular Problems in Musculoskeletal Disorders of the Limbs

1981. 98 figures. X, 404 pages
ISBN 3-540-90524-3

Written in clear, clinical language, this is the only book devoted exclusively to vascular complications in orthopaedics.
The basic scientific foundations – anatomy, physiology, and pathophysiology of circulation in the bones, joints, skin, and voluntary muscles of the limbs – needed to make an accurate differential diagnosis are thoroughly examined. Physical and laboratory tests used to diagnose vascular disorders that may hinder orthopaedic conditions are presented in detail. Vascular complications are approached from every possible angle: vascular manifestations common to both circulatory and orthopaedic conditions, vascular findings which mimic orthopaedic conditions, vascular complications of therapeutic orthopaedic procedures, and vascular complications induced by trauma.
In addition, the legal implications of treatment are considered, along with topics of current interest such as limb replantation and compartment syndromes.

A. Wackenheim

Cheirolumbar Dysostosis

Developmental Brachycheiry and Stenosis of the Bony Vertebral Lumbar Canal
With collaboration of E. Babin, P. Bourjat, E. Bromhorst, R. M. Kipper, R. Ludwiczak, G. Vetter
Translated from the French by M. I. Wackenheim
1980. 39 figures, 85 tables. VII, 102 pages
ISBN 3-540-10371-6

Developmental stenosis of the vertebral canal is a condition that had gone unnoticed until the pioneering efforts of H. Verbiest alerted the medical profession to its existence. This neglect, moreover, hindered research into its causes and possible association with other dysostoses.
In this monograph, the author builds upon the work of his colleague to describe the association of the hypertrophic form of ideopathic developmental stenosis of the lumbar vertebral canal with developmental brachyphalangia, brachymetacarpia, or a combination of both. The conclusive evidence for this new disease entity, called cheirolumbar dysostosis, is provided in the extensive study of 29 patients. The author carefully describes the various types of brachyphalangia and brachymetacarpia and presents in tabular form normal values for phalangeal and metacarpal lengths. After discussing the anomalies exhibited in the patients' lumbar vertebral canals and hands, the author concludes with a consideration of the genetic factors involved in the disease's transmission.
This monograph will prove invaluable to physicians and researchers involved in the field of spinal abnormalities, alerting them to signs present in other skeletal parts of the body.

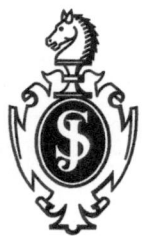

Springer-Verlag
Berlin
Heidelberg
New York